D0986306

2012

Maximum
HEALING

Maximum HEALING

Optimize Your Natural Ability to Heal

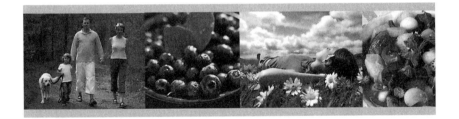

H. ROBERT SILVERSTEIN, MD, FACC

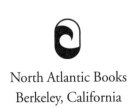

North Atlantic Books
Berkeley, California

Published by
North Atlantic Books
P.O. Box 12327
Berkeley, California 94712

Cover and book design by Suzanne Albertson
Cover images © iStockphoto.com/Wojciech Gajda; iStockphoto.com/Joe Biafore; iStockphoto.com/ALEAIMAGE; iStockphoto.com/Elzbieta Sekowska
Printed in the United States of America

Maximum Healing: Optimize Your Natural Ability to Heal is sponsored by the Society for the Study of Native Arts and Sciences, a nonprofit educational corporation whose goals are to develop an educational and cross-cultural perspective linking various scientific, social, and artistic fields; to nurture a holistic view of arts, sciences, humanities, and healing; and to publish and distribute literature on the relationship of mind, body, and nature.

North Atlantic Books' publications are available through most bookstores. For further information, visit our website at www.northatlanticbooks.com or call 800-733-3000.

MEDICAL DISCLAIMER: The following information is intended for general information purposes only. Individuals should always see their health care provider before administering any suggestions made in this book. Any application of the material set forth in the following pages is at the reader's discretion and is his or her sole responsibility.

Library of Congress Cataloging-in-Publication Data
Silverstein, H. Robert.
    Maximum healing : optimize your natural ability to heal / H. Robert Silverstein.
        p. cm.
    Summary: "Combining conventional Western and holistic medical approaches, Maximum Healing presents a complete guide to improving the immune system including a thirty-day program designed to reestablish health through diet, exercise, and stress reduction"—Provided by publisher.
        ISBN 978-1-55643-922-3
    1. Immunity—Nutritional aspects. 2. Holistic medicine. 3. Alternative medicine. 4. Healing. 5. Health. I. Title.
    QR182.2.N86S55 2010
    616.07'9—dc22
                                                    2010000621

1 2 3 4 5 6 7 8 9 SHERIDAN 14 13 12 11 10

This book is dedicated to all who strive with, or against, the current of what seems to be common knowledge and usual behaviors. It is truly dedicated to Denis Burkitt, Nathan Pritikin, Bill Spear, and Dean Ornish, MD, who saw that most diseases have preventable or correctable origins, when viewed through the lens of what are the basic requirements of our human biology.

Acknowledgments

Maximum Healing is a collaborative effort that would not have come to fruition without the help of talented, dedicated, and highly skilled people.

First and foremost, I wish to thank Tom Monte, an established and sought-after medical writer and researcher, for providing much of the scientific data and the literary approach for this work. His efforts serve as an effective backdrop to the anecdotal evidence of the healing successes of many of my patients.

I wish to acknowledge my patients for continually inspiring me. I am their enthusiastic partner in the quest to optimize their innate ability to heal. Although the case histories in this book are inspired by actual events or a combination of patient events, patient names have been changed in order to protect patient privacy and doctor-patient confidentiality.

Thanks to Elizabeth W. Preston, MA, for her computer and formatting skills as well as Jacqueline John. I wish to thank Diane Dadiskos, MS, (a patient who has been cancer-free for six years) for her creativity, unbridled enthusiasm, strength, persistence, and, repeatedly, the finest judgment in facilitating the publication of this work.

Lastly, none of this would have been possible were it not for Jill and her sister Jackie, my office managers, who maintained my busy office practice while all the "meshugas" of writing this book was happening.

Contents

"A fully functional immune system is essential for self-preservation and good health."

—ROBERT C. CARTER, MD,
Mayo Clinic Proceedings, March 2006, 81 (3): 337–384

"This is a return to the common sense (of) holistic . . . natural healing by correcting . . . mistakes of living."

—HAROLD KALUNGIAN, MA,
"New Holistic Paradigm for Natural Healing," 2006

"Most diseases occur if, and only if, the person with a genetic tendency does what is necessary to express that genetic tendency. While people have the 'tendency' to high cholesterol, high blood pressure, diabetes, cancer of the breast, diverticulitis, gallstones, etc., these diseases occur if, and only if, these susceptible people do what is necessary to cause the expression of that genetic tendency/disease. In that sense, all diseases are 'genetic' and merely represent the interaction of that person's genetic tendency coming in contact with a specific (and disease generating) behavior, very much as a lighted match plus gasoline creates fire."

—H. ROBERT SILVERSTEIN, MD, FACC

Foreword

What is it about this book that makes me, a very busy, practicing board-certified pulmonary specialist, conclude that its messages are extremely important and demand our very careful attention? Also, what is it about this book that made me ponder the fact that I have probably been off course regarding how I have managed the care of my patients for the past twenty-seven years? It is time for me to confront the uncomfortable truth about what I have been doing every day on the job.

I consider myself a typical American doctor practicing traditional Western medicine. I've taken care of thousands of patients the best way I know how, and I almost never questioned my methods or my beliefs because that's the way I have been taught. I always thought that the actions that I have been trained to carry out must be correct because science says so. My teachers told me so. The medical journals told me so. And drug companies told me so. Patients believed in my methods. And I was smart enough to get into medical school! So of course, we doctors must all be right about what we've been doing in healthcare for decades.

We American physicians emerged in an era in which we were trained to "fix things that were broken." It's our way now. From the time we enter medical school, we learn about diseases, what causes them, their appearances under the microscope, the biochemistry and microbiology of damage, and then we are trained to "do things" that will make the damage go away. If we can't treat with medicines, we try to operate the damage away with bypasses or resections. Or burn it away with radiation, or poison it away with chemotherapy. It's how we've done things in the Western medical model for decades. In fact, the responsibility for illness has frequently been thought of as the fault of the patient and not the physician.

So, really, the question that confronts medical practice in the new millennium now and that needs our most careful attention is just this: Do we American physicians really do everything we can do to fix the problems facing health care in America? And at least in my mind, and certainly in Dr. Silverstein's book, you will find that the answer has to be a resounding ... "NO."

Let's consider that there exist three entirely different populations of patients who seek health care in America. First, there are the ill patients who want treatment for an illness that has already manifested itself. Second, there are the patients with conditions such as obesity, hypertension, diabetes, inflammatory bowel disease, or high cholesterol who need modification in their lives before they become ill. And third, there are the healthy, usually younger Americans who want to stay that way and not accumulate the conditions that would lead to illness or damage to their bodies as they get older.

Doctors in America concentrate on the first population for the vast majority of their time. But, what about the others? Dr. Silverstein, in his book, *Maximum Healing,* focuses on the second and third populations of patients and this is the magic that has developed through his years of experience. He focuses on the prevention of illness before it happens. This is the correct way. Not the way I've been practicing health care for almost three decades. And it is my firm belief that this is exactly where Western medical practitioners need to focus if we are to do the job we committed ourselves to do since medical school: promote health and wellness. We have been misdirected for so long.

This book is essentially a comprehensive prescription for better health for everyone. But at the same time, Dr. Silverstein recognizes that each person is an individual with highly personal characteristics that make our conditions unique. There are modifications in our lifestyle that we can all do to help improve our health. And, there are also actions that are specific to the individual patient's condition that can help to achieve better results. In this respect, the information presented here is not simply a quick gimmick to better health.

I think that diet modification is the first and most important step to good health. After all, "we are what we eat," aren't we? Diet modification is also hardest of all to achieve because the foods that are considered bad for us taste the best and are the most readily accessible. Few people question anymore that the fast food revolution over the past several decades has been largely responsible for the obesity crisis we face today. But this is where we need to start and Dr. Silverstein properly focuses on this important component of good health and the way to prevent disease from happening in the first place. Grains, vegetables, beans, some fresh fruits, nuts, and seeds are the building blocks; so that is where you start and how to do it is covered very well in these pages.

The role of supplements as a way to boost immunity is also presented and from a research point of view, we are completely at the infancy of knowledge concerning what is the best combination of herbs, antioxidants, and vitamins to give us the best results. The information contained here is a wonderful start to get to where we should be. Considering the natural benefit we see with supplement use so far, I am encouraged that supplements, in addition to healthy diet modification, are the right course for the future as well.

Finally, there are guidelines for not only eating well and adding supplements to the mix, but also for living life successfully in order to promote good health *for the distance.* No one would argue that clean air and water make sense. But clear air also means not smoking, and this behavior must be incorporated into the overall picture if the best results are to come out of Dr. Silverstein's recommendations. And everyone would agree that exercise is a wonderful thing to do. But how many of us make the excuse that we just couldn't get to the gym today or take that thirty-minute walk in the neighborhood that we said we would.

The responsibility isn't on the doctor or the patient alone anymore, but on both. Good health is a true partnership. Wellness before illness strikes requires important modifications in how both the doctor and the patient have been doing things for years. Both need to change. It requires the education for us to know what we are supposed to do and then it requires motivation to get the job done. It is a team collaboration with the doctor promoting the best education possible and the patient willing to stop bad habits and incorporate new healthy habits for the long run. It's the only way now. And I plan to change the way I've been doing things for decades.

MICHAEL B. TEIGER, MD, FCCP

Foreword

Medical school education in the 1970s focused almost exclusively on the diagnosis and treatment of disease processes. While it was recognized that tobacco, excessive alcohol consumption, obesity, and sedentary lifestyle were potentially harmful to our health, little emphasis was placed on dealing with the prevention of illness. Treatment was generally not oriented towards changing the behaviors that were responsible for generating these disease states.

It was in the fall of 1992 when I first met Dr. Silverstein. I was experiencing what seemed to be an elevated discharge of catecholamines that was evidenced by irregular heartbeats, elevated blood pressure and heart rate, and anxiety. Dr. Silverstein easily diagnosed the problem and following a thorough workup, he explained the etiology of my symptoms, and more importantly, changes in lifestyle that had the potential to resolve this problem and prevent recurrence.

Choosing to see Dr. Silverstein was anything but random. I had heard of his work and was searching for an approach that was different from the standard fare. A number of my colleagues, predictably, had told me to "consume less caffeine, work less intensely, and get more sleep." While these recommendations were helpful, they seemed insufficient. During my eighteen-year association with Dr. Silverstein, we have become not only close medical colleagues but also the best of friends. We share a number of patients, have developed close family ties, and frequently discuss the latest advances in our respective specialties.

While we all respect the researchers who constantly add knowledge and direction to the teaching and practice of medicine, I am most amazed by the pioneers who literally break new ground. H. Robert Silverstein, MD, is such a pioneer. His theories on diet, cholesterol metabolism, and blood pressure regulation were at least a decade ahead of the curve.

It has been a privilege to be his friend, colleague, and in many ways his student.

LAURENCE GOLDSTEIN, MD, Senior attending, Department of Psychiatry, Hartford Hospital, Hartford, Connecticut

Introduction

For the past twenty-five years, I have been combining modern, conventional Western medical approaches with complementary medicine, such as diet, supplements and herbs, and exercise. I am a board-certified Cardiologist and Internist and the Medical Director of the Preventive Medicine Center in Hartford, Connecticut. I am a member of the medical staffs at St. Francis and Hartford Hospitals. I am also Clinical Assistant Professor of Medicine at the University of Connecticut School of Medicine. Most of my time is spent treating people in the Hartford area who come to my office suffering from virtually every illness imaginable. In the majority of cases, I use conventional Western medicine as well as natural healing methods to treat my patients. Very often, I find that natural healing methods alone are sufficient to restore health, even when people are suffering from a long history of illness or have used conventional medical treatments unsuccessfully. I call my approach CAIM or Complementary-Alternative-Integrative-Medicine. Essentially, my program combines and integrates modern medical practices with alternative and ancient forms of healing. In this book, I will show you how to incorporate natural healing methods to improve every aspect of your health.

Whenever we explore the relative strength or weakness of the human immune system, we run up against a single pivotal factor: *you*. To be more specific, your behavior—how you live your life—interacts with your genetic or biologically learned makeup and affects your susceptibility to illness. In a great many instances, your behavior determines whether or not you will become ill; whether you will fully recover; and how strong your immune function will be when you do.

This central issue of lifestyle behavior management is one of the big differences between conventional Western medicine and the more complementary or integrative healing approaches.

In complementary or integrative medicine, physician and patient are coworkers toward the same end: making the patient well. The physician who uses natural medicine is both a healer and a teacher. The doctor offers foods, herbs, and nutritional supplements as medicines, but he or she also relies on the patient to make progressively well-considered lifestyle changes designed to eradicate the origins of disease as well as to boost the body's own healing powers—namely, the immune system.

Far too often in the U.S. health care system, medical doctors prescribe medicines designed to eradicate signs or symptoms, without asking and adequately educating the patient to change the very behaviors that have caused the underlying illness.

When we view health and illness through the lens of the human immune system, so to speak, we realize that virtually all major illnesses we deal with today result when toxic substances, hormones, and foreign chemicals accumulate within the body and often trigger an immune reaction that we typically refer to as inflammation. That word, coined by the Greeks to mean "a fire within," occurs when the body is overcome with poorly tolerated unnatural substances from our diet, environment, and lifestyle along with consistently harmful emotions.

The impact of these accumulating and progressively toxic influences depresses the immune (and every other) system and makes us more vulnerable to disease. Eventually, we get sick with anything from the common cold or flu to more serious illnesses. In a great many cases, the illness is self-created. Now I am not implying that the majority of patients are hypochondriacs. I am saying that personal choice in diet, exercise, and lifestyle has a huge effect on health.

As twentieth-century history has demonstrated, medicines and surgery have limited effectiveness when it comes to treating these illnesses. In my experience, I have found behavioral changes, sometimes coupled with medical advice or interventions as in integrative medicine rather than conventional medicine or surgery alone, to be much more effective. When the toxins, for lack of a better word, are removed and immune-boosting nutrients and herbal and supplemental remedies are added, even the most devastating illnesses can often be overcome, as I demonstrate here in *Maximum Healing*.

As you read this book, you'll learn how to strengthen your immune systems and restore your health. You can overcome nagging colds, allergies, asthma, weight gain, and many forms of chronic disease, including heart disease, diabetes, and other degenerative illnesses. In the following pages, you'll read some remarkable case histories for every illness, includ-ing cancer.

The book is written in the first person in easy-to-understand language. Working with medical writer Tom Monte, who has a long and proven track record writing medical articles and books, helped me to do that.

Maximum Healing combines a modern scientific approach with my experience using natural healing techniques, giving readers an advanced form of integrative medicine. It is an optimal model for twenty-first cen-tury healthcare. I hope you will find the program presented here to be enlightening and helpful. I believe that you can vastly improve the qual-ity of your life by following the principles of *Maximum Healing,* while living longer and enjoying life to the fullest.

PART I

Understanding Your Immune System

CHAPTER ONE

The Crossroads: A Choice Between Health and Illness

Here is a startling fact: more people today suffer from immune-related disorders than at any other time in human history.

And it's no wonder.

Your body's defenses are assaulted by a tidal wave of toxins that travel through the air, water, and food, or develop from everyday behaviors, many of which you take for granted. Our current lifestyles are stretching our immune systems to their limits. Toxins in our foods, air, water, and soil are making you—and everyone else—more vulnerable to disease than ever before.

The consequences of such conditions are disease epidemics. Asthma, diabetes, and cancer are all increasing in unprecedented numbers. Heart disease, very much an immune/inflammatory-related disorder, remains the leading killer disease in the world today. At the same time, non-life-threatening diseases are rising at alarming rates as well. These include allergies, skin disorders, joint pain, headaches, backaches, chronic fevers, muscle tension, and nervous system disorders. If you suffer from any of these major or minor health issues, the chances are excellent that your immune system is seriously impaired.

I have been practicing medicine for thirty years, and in that time, I have witnessed a steady decline in the general health of my patients. I have been especially struck by the declining strength of their immune defenses. This observation, coupled with the successes I have witnessed with my Maximum Healing Program, is what drove me to write this book.

Over the last three decades, I have watched as younger and younger people arrive in my office with illnesses that I used to think of as diseases of maturity and old age. Diabetes, arthritis, and heart disease are but three examples of disorders that are affecting young people as never before. These are inflammatory diseases, in large part, that stem from overstressed and weakened immune systems. Other immune-related problems are also on the rise: asthma, allergies, inflammatory bowel disorders (including Crohn's disease and colitis), eczema, dermatitis, and rosacea. Very often, these diseases may be harbingers of more severe illnesses, including cancers of the breast, colon, and prostate, as well as coronary heart disease.

The remarkable truth is that most of these diseases are preventable, even curable, if patients are willing to make a few modifications to their diet and lifestyle. The addition of certain foods, supplements, herbs, and immune-boosting behaviors can dramatically strengthen your immune defenses and help you to virtually overcome many illnesses.

Most of us fail to realize just how powerful our immune systems really are. Consider, for a moment, the fact that a healthy adult produces anywhere from two hundred and fifty thousand to five hundred thousand cancer cells each day. That's a frightening thought, I know, but the body is more than capable of wiping out the early stages of this terrifying disease. Again, it is your immune system—along with various cancer-fighting mechanisms that I will talk about in this book—that comes to your rescue. Even cancer, one of the most dreaded of all diseases, is inferior to the onslaught of this incredible defense system that is alive in each of us. That is, provided your system is working properly.

Humans cannot survive without a strong immune system.

What most of us don't realize is that our daily behavior determines the strength of our immune defenses. It also determines, to a great extent, our body's capacity to heal and overcome illness.

The human body has miraculous healing powers. Those healing powers can overcome illnesses; even those that we have long believed were incurable. Very often, we don't have to make enormous changes in our diet and lifestyle in order to provide our bodies with the right conditions to heal.

Sharon is a good example of the kinds of changes I'm talking about. She was twenty-eight years old when she first came to see me, suffering from asthma and an array of conditions that included hay fever, joint pain, and chronic headaches. She had chronic fatigue syndrome and was about twenty pounds overweight. At the time, Sharon was taking three medications for her asthma, all by inhaler. The first was Advair, a steroid with a long-acting form of albuterol to reduce inflammation. The second was a fast-acting form of albuterol, to relax the bronchial muscles and promote easier breathing. The third was Spiriva, a drug that relaxes the bronchial passages. These were state-of-the-art medications for asthma. In addition, Sharon had been taking a variety of over-the-counter drugs for her allergies, though she had not been having much success with any of them. Her symptoms persisted, especially during the spring and fall.

I ran a standard array of blood tests on Sharon, took a medical and a dietary history, and did a complete physical exam. I found that, by conventional standards, her diet was pretty good. She ate a wide variety of grains and grain products, vegetables, fish, soy products, some chicken, red meat, and a good deal of yogurt. I told her that we could rotate through different medications for her asthma and allergies, but I had a feeling that—as far as the medication was concerned—we weren't going to do much better than what she was taking.

Instead, I asked Sharon if she would adopt a program that included dietary changes, the addition of a few supplements (to be taken periodically), and changes in lifestyle. These changes in behavior, I suggested, could reduce her symptoms and, if we were lucky, eliminate them altogether. Sharon said she was willing to give the program a try.

The first thing I recommended was that, for now, she eliminate three foods from her diet: all forms of milk, including skim milk, cheese, and yogurt; all foods containing wheat, including wheat bread and wheat-containing pastas; and all soy products, including tofu. (These recommendations are part of the Maximum Healing Diet, which I describe in Chapter Ten.)

I explained that many people suffer allergic reactions to these three foods, especially to dairy products. The immune system recognizes the dairy proteins as "not-self," meaning the body responds to dairy products as a foreign substance that represents a threat to health. Once that recognition is made, immune cells attack the dairy proteins—but they frequently attack normal, healthy tissues with a similar molecular structure, or start a cascade of biochemical changes, as well. At that point, a full-scale immune reaction can occur. Such an immune-triggered attack generates inflammation. That attack, and subsequent inflammatory reaction, can be launched against connective tissue in the joints, as well as against tissues in the bronchial passages, lungs, large intestine, and other organs.

Children are often especially sensitive to dairy proteins. Allergists are well aware that dairy foods (milk and milk products) can sometimes cause chronic runny nose, iron loss, ear infections, and a variety of other allergic reactions, including headaches, sore throats, and recurrent upper respiratory tract infections. In addition to dairy proteins, there is also the question of lactose, the sugar in milk products, which many adults (especially people of color) cannot tolerate.

In my experience, I have found that taking people with asthma, or any allergy, off dairy products frequently brings about a partial or complete relief from all symptoms. But I couldn't be sure that Sharon was just allergic to dairy foods. Many people are often sensitive to the protein and fiber in wheat products, as well as the proteins in soy. I have found that removing these foods from the diets of people with allergies (or bowel disease) often results in a diminution or clearance of symptoms. Instead of wheat bread and standard noodles, I told Sharon that she could eat rice or spelt bread and rice or quinoa pasta, both of which are wheat-free.

In addition to these changes, I placed Sharon on a food-based supplement, called One Daily, a product of MegaFood that provides a wide spectrum of vitamins and minerals. The nutrients in the supplement are extremely easy to assimilate because they are in the form in which they exist in foods. I also added the MegaFood Antioxidant formula.

I asked Sharon to take these nutrients on Monday, Tuesday, Thursday, and Friday, and abstain on "Wednesdays and the Weekends Off" or what I like to call "WWO." I do not recommend taking supplements every day, nor do I believe that they should be taken indefinitely. I recommended that she take them for three months, which would significantly boost her immune system. During that time, we would monitor her health and adjust the program if needed. Occasionally I use and recommend Moducare for misguided immune reactions.

These changes caused a remarkable transformation in Sharon's condition. After a few weeks, her asthma and allergy symptoms diminished significantly. Her energy levels rose dramatically, and she began losing weight. Sharon and I worked together to reduce her medication, and six months later she no longer needed daily doses of her asthma medication. Instead, she needed only a rare dose of her albuterol inhaler. As for her allergies, they cleared up entirely; she no longer needed allergy medication. She also lost fifteen pounds and naturally kept the weight off.

For Sharon, these improvements were life changing, but I have found that such improvements in health can almost always be predicted. In fact, given the right circumstances, your immune system can—and often does—overcome just about anything.

Sharon is one of thousands of people whom I have successfully treated with the Maximum Healing Program I describe in this book—a program that consists primarily of dietary change, exercise, herbs, supplements, and other modifications in lifestyle.

As you will read, this program can dramatically boost the healing forces in your body and help you overcome many forms of illness. In most cases, people will begin to see dramatic results within two weeks, and certainly within thirty days of adopting my approach. Like the people I describe in this book, the program can help you overcome intractable, and in some cases even life-threatening diseases.

Each of Us Has Unique Vulnerabilities

Experiences with people like Sharon have taught me that each of us has our own unique sensitivities. In fact, I have yet to meet the person who does not have his or her own set of personal vulnerabilities to food substances, chemicals, and emotional and psychological states.

If you are going to optimize your immune system and enjoy all the benefits of good health, you must learn to reflect on how food and other areas of your life are affecting you personally. Just because everyone else appears to be okay when they drink milk or eat cheese, soy products, or wheat, that doesn't necessarily mean that your body can tolerate such foods. I can't tell you how many patients have said to me, "But Doc"—and I hate being called "Doc"; it's either "Robert" or "Doctor"—"everyone eats these foods, and they seem to be fine. Why can't I eat them and be fine, too?"

In fact, everyone isn't fine. As a population, we are becoming increasingly sensitive, and therefore vulnerable, to the Standard American Diet (SAD) as a whole, and particularly to certain substances within the diet. SAD is rich in processed foods and high in sugar, salt, and fat. These substances can have a profound effect on our biology, transforming healthy cells into diseased ones.

Many people suffer from illnesses that appear to result from an immune system that has run amuck—that is, their system has turned against them. There are myriad such diseases, but the most common autoimmune diseases are allergies, rheumatoid arthritis, type I juvenile diabetes, multiple sclerosis, and systemic lupus erythematosus (SLE).

Autoimmune diseases appear to be the ultimate form of biological self-destruction. They occur when our immune defenses become unbalanced. The immune defenses turn against us, causing an array of consequences: everything from mild physical distress to life-threatening diseases. In such cases, we appear to be innocent victims of a biology gone wrong. But there may be more to the autoimmune story than we think. In some cases, we may be introducing substances into the body that are actually causing disease states. Two such disorders, type 1 juvenile diabetes and rheumatoid arthritis, are good examples of what I am talking about.

Scientists at Johns Hopkins University found that cow's milk can trigger the onset of type 1 juvenile diabetes in sensitive children. Reporting their work in the *New England Journal of Medicine* (July 1992), researchers found that children produced antibodies in response to proteins in cow's milk, specifically bovine albumin peptide. The antibodies to the cow's milk proteins attached themselves to the beta cells of the pancreas. The beta cells of the pancreas produce insulin. The antibodies from the cow's milk protein attacked and destroyed the beta cells.

Insulin is the hormone used by the body to make sugar available to cells. Without insulin, blood sugar rises, but this sugar cannot get into the cells to nourish them, and the cells die. In the Johns Hopkins study, the antibodies that attacked the pancreatic beta cell proteins probably destroyed them. This, of course, destroyed the pancreas' ability to produce insulin, resulting in type 1 diabetes.

Scientists have known for many years that childhood diabetes was caused by an immune response that destroyed insulin-producing cells. Animal studies have shown that cow's milk can trigger that autoimmune reaction and cause diabetes. Moreover, researchers have found that diabetes turns up in wealthy populations that consume large quantities of dairy products. Conversely, it is rare in populations that do not consume cow's milk, such as those in Asia and Africa. Researchers have also found that feeding infants only breast milk not only delays the consumption of milk products, but also reduces the risk of childhood diabetes (*New England Journal of Medicine* 1992, 327:302–7)

Another autoimmune disorder is rheumatoid arthritis, a very painful condition in which the immune system attacks and deforms tissues in the joints. Several studies, including research published in the British medical journal *Lancet* (October 12, 1991) and the *American Journal of Clinical Nutrition* (May 2000), have shown that fasting, followed by a vegetarian diet, significantly improves the symptoms associated with rheumatoid arthritis.

Norwegian researcher J. Kjekdsen-Kragh and his coworkers found that seven to ten days of fasting, followed by four weeks of an individually-adjusted, gluten-free, vegan diet caused "significant improvement in the number of tender joints, Ritchie's articular index, [the] number of swollen joints, pain score, duration of morning stiffness, grip strength," and a wide array of blood factors related to arthritis, including "erythrocyte sedimentation rate, C-reactive protein, and white blood cell count."

The people involved in the study also experienced remarkable improvements in their overall health. Many rheumatologists that I have encountered are aware of this information but still don't act on it.

Other studies have shown that dairy products are linked with an increase in inflammatory arthritis, which is common in dairy-consuming Western nations, such as the United States, Canada, Europe, Australia, and New Zealand. Reading study after study on the effect of animal proteins on the human immune system, it's very possible to conclude that one of the primary causes of arthritis is an immune reaction caused by the presence of certain animal protein portions (peptides) in the blood, especially proteins from dairy foods. Once animal proteins/peptides make their way into the blood of sensitive people, the immune system produces antibodies whose mission is to attack and destroy these proteins. These proteins combine with antibodies to form compounds called "immune complexes." These immune complexes take up residence in the joints and act as irritants, much the same way a sliver of wood irritates your finger when you get a splinter.

The answer to many of these problems may be to eliminate particular animal proteins. I recommend a total elimination of dairy foods. However, not all animal proteins may adversely affect you.

This is the question that arises when we look at both of these illnesses a little more closely: is it possible that we are introducing substances into the body that individual people are prone to react to due to a unique vulnerability or genetic predisposition? Is it possible that each of us has individual limits when it comes to certain foods and nutrients? I believe so.

After thirty years as a medical doctor, I have found that some people cannot eat dairy foods without suffering an array of symptoms. Others have trouble with spices, chocolate, wheat products, or soy protein. This is not the case for everyone; some people are fine drinking milk products or eating a little chocolate. But for sensitive people—and there are many more than we realize—these foods appear to trigger an immune reaction that results in various disorders.

It's very possible that current environmental conditions, which include air, water, and food, are themselves severely immune-depressing. Under such conditions, many of us are becoming increasingly sensitive to certain substances, such as the proteins in milk products, wheat, or soy. These are just a few substances that trigger these destructive reactions among an increasing number of people today.

The Five Keys to Health

To protect yourself from disease, you must reduce the overall toxic burden on your immune system. To do that, you must improve the quality of your life in five key areas.

It is no exaggeration to say that how you behave in these five areas of your life determines the quality of your health.

The five critical domains that affect your immune system and, ultimately, your health, are:

1. The quality of the *air* you breathe
2. The quality of the *water* you drink
3. The quality of the *food* you eat
4. The degree of physical *activity* you engage in
5. The degree of positive *feelings* and stability in your psychological and emotional life

Domain One: The Air You Breathe

Many of you live in cities, where you have little or no control of the air quality in your environment. That is all the more reason to avoid smoking cigarettes and to stay away from secondhand smoke. If the air you are breathing is already polluted, don't add to it.

Your body can tolerate a certain amount of toxicity in all five domains, but everyone has limits. I have found that if you act wisely in three or four domains, excesses in the other one or two are more easily tolerated.

Cigarette smoking can negate all the good you do in other areas of your life. If you cannot quit the smoking habit, consider using Sun Pure or Airex Model 45 air filters. They may be a bit expensive, but well worth it to give you cleaner air. Do not buy air filters that emit ozone.

Domain Two: The Water You Drink

Water is the basis for all the liquids in your body. Water-based liquids in your body include your tissue fluid, lymph, mucous, and urine. Water bathes and lubricates your joints and eyes. It is the basis for saliva and for sweat, which eliminates toxins through the skin. Like air, water is essential for life. Good, clean, pure water is essential for good health. I don't recommend water from plastic bottles.

The first thing we have to realize when considering water is that it must be clean. Unfortunately, there are a lot of toxins in our water supply, including arsenic, chlorine, asbestos, cadmium, lead, and nitrate, as well as many pathogenic microorganisms.

It's essential to improve the quality of the water you drink. You probably should drink more water in order to help improve digestion, bowel function, and assimilation of nutrients.

Here's my recommendation for improving your water quality immediately: Sip filtered water or weak tea throughout the day at your desk, or at home. Have a glass or metal water bottle of water in your car and sip some as you drive. Water cleanses the system of so many toxins. It's a simple change you can make. My preferred water filtering system is the Nikken. As you increase your consumption of pure water, you should decrease your consumption of toxic liquids such as alcohol, juices, coffee, and soft drinks, which affect the workings of the immune system and our overall health. However, nothing is totally prohibited as a general rule.

Domain Three: The Foods You Eat
—A Liv-it (not a Die-t)

Humans are genetically engineered predominantly as a plant-eating species. Our salivary glands contain the enzyme ptyalin for digesting carbohydrates. We have a long small bowel (twelve body lengths) like plant-eating animals such as goats and gorillas, not a short small bowel (three body lengths) like carnivores, such as dogs, tigers, and crocodiles. Our teeth are flat to grind vegetarian food, not scissor-like to tear meat. We do not have fangs and claws, like carnivores. We do have four poorly developed canine teeth—out of thirty-two total teeth in our mouths—to eat meat. Four canine teeth out of thirty-two teeth translates to one out of eight meals, or optimally eating meat once every three days or twice a week. The optimal serving size is equivalent to the size of the palm of the individual doing the eating.

Foods high in cholesterol do not raise the blood cholesterol of carnivorous meat eaters but will raise the blood cholesterol of vegetarian animals like humans.

We coevolved over approximately two million years with the plant kingdom. There is such a thing as a human diet—a way of eating what the body was designed to eat, a way of eating that supports our biology. I call it "The Natural Human Design."

Our ancient ancestors ate a diet that came directly from nature. I refer to this diet as "The Food Mantra": fresh fruits and vegetables, whole and unprocessed grains and beans, ideally organic, and made up of at least 90 percent fiber.

The Food Mantra diet of our ancestors was not stripped of nutrients or adulterated by artificial chemicals. There were no synthetic foods. The animal foods consumed back then were wild, low in total fat, low in saturated fat, and high in beneficial omega-3 fats. Of course, current environmental toxins did not affect early humans.

The consequence of living within those dietary limits was—and, for many people, still is—good health. This is the case even for people who live according to their traditional ways today, such as the !Kung tribe of Botswana. As a tribe, the !Kung have the same percentage of people living to the age of sixty and older as do contemporary Americans. And yet, they live without medical tests, checkups, pharmaceutical drugs, or surgery.

If a member of the !Kung community does not die of an accident or an infectious disease early in life, he or she enjoys a better chance of living to old age than a Westerner. The Tarahumara Indians of Northern Mexico are another example of a traditional people who enjoy remarkably good health. They have exceedingly low rates of heart disease, cancer, adult-onset diabetes, obesity, arthritis, and other serious illnesses. They eat a diet made up largely of whole grains, fresh vegetables, fruit, fish, and small amounts of red meat. Meat is eaten as a condiment. All of this makes their diets extremely rich in nutrition but very low in saturated fats. They eat no processed synthetic food, which means they consume no trans-fatty acids. Trans-fatty acids—often referred to as hydrogenated fats—have been shown to increase your risk of heart disease, diabetes, and cancer.

In 1989, after studying the health and dietary patterns of six thousand five hundred families living in China, Dr. T. Colin Campbell, a nutritionist and biochemist at Cornell University, wrote *The China Study,* which has been hailed as one of the most comprehensive studies of nutrition ever conducted. Dr. Campbell found that the best predictor of whether or not a Chinese person would suffer a serious illness was his or her blood cholesterol level.

"So far we've seen that plasma cholesterol is a good predictor of the kinds of diseases people are going to get," Dr. Campbell told the *New York Times.* "Those with higher cholesterol levels are prone to diseases of affluence—cancer, heart disease, osteoporosis, and diabetes. We're basically a vegetarian species and should be eating a wide variety of plant foods and minimizing our intake of animal foods."

The current modern diet—rich in processed foods, sweets, salt, and fat—is an aberration, at least in terms of human experience. It is unlike anything we have ever seen, much less eaten before. This modern diet is extremely poisonous to our biology and, specifically, to our immune systems.

I have developed a way of eating (which I call the **Liv-it**, rather than a die-t) that can profoundly improve your health. In the pages that follow, I will show you how to gradually change your current eating habits so that you can easily and smoothly adopt my delicious and satisfying immune-boosting eating plan.

Domain Four: The Exercise You Engage In—Or Avoid

Humans are designed to be physically active and free of excess fat. Our lack of activity, coupled with a diet rich in fat and processed carbohydrates, has resulted in an epidemic of obesity. Not only has this diet affected the adult population; it is destroying the lives of many young children. Excess body weight caused from consuming high-fat foods, as I will show, is weakening our immune systems and giving rise to a wide array of inflammatory diseases, including coronary heart disease, cancer, high blood pressure, and diabetes.

Domain Five: The Thoughts You Think

I believe the quality of your thoughts directly affects your overall health. You must find ways to think positively and to experience and express positive thoughts and emotions, not out of altruism, but for your own good.

Negative thoughts have a profound effect on your physical body. They create tremendous fear, anxiety, muscle tension, hormonal imbalances, and changes in respiration, heart rate, and brain function. Positive thoughts have exactly the opposite effect: they cause deeper levels of physical relaxation, the reduction of muscle tension, a more balanced hormonal environment, deeper and fuller respiration, and improved heart and brain function.

If You Want to Be Well, You Must Do More

We have distinct limits as to how much pollution we can safely take in from our air, water, food, thinking, and emotional life. We are required by our natural design to engage in physical activity and experience deep and restful sleep if we are to be healthy. If we live outside the limits of our Natural Human Design (what people are biologically designed to take in and do), we become sick. Eventually, we can become seriously ill and die prematurely.

Today we are essentially abusing ourselves in these five critical domains of life—breathing, drinking, eating, exercise, and thinking. And, in the process, we are becoming increasingly dependent upon doctors, medication, and surgery.

Most of us take this dependency for granted. Your doctor can only do so much, however. The power to radically transform your health is in your hands.

Nothing in your body illustrates this better than your immune system. Aside from giving you a vaccine, your doctor can do little to boost your immune function. On the other hand, you can do a great deal to strengthen your defenses. The changes you make can mean the difference between health and sickness, and even life and death. Allow me to give you a short example.

In 2002, I was presented with the Community Service Award given by the International Society for Hypertension in Blacks (ISHIB), an award I was very honored to receive. About half of my patients, many of whom suffer from high blood pressure, are from the minority community in Hartford. I have had a great deal of success treating that disease, in part because the lifestyle changes that I encourage can have a profound effect on hypertension. But the truth is, the award that I was given was more a result of what my patients did for themselves, than from what I did for them.

A doctor can do three things when it comes to treating high blood pressure: prescribe medication; teach the person which lifestyle changes to make and why those changes are so important; and encourage the patient to adopt these changes and maintain them over time. Medications should be considered a short-term treatment, especially because they may have many unwanted side effects. But lifestyle changes, especially in diet and exercise, can bring about a significant reduction in weight, lower blood cholesterol, improved circulation and cardiovascular function, and lower blood pressure. In a great many cases, these changes can restore normal blood pressure and free a person from all medication.

Ultimately it is all about freedom. In fact, I refer to myself as an "abolitionist physician." I am for the abolition of diseases.

Blood pressure is not the only aspect of health that these changes will affect, however. Virtually every part of a person's life improves. Who is responsible for making those changes? In the early stages, the doctor is essential for prescribing appropriate medication and coaching a person to make the right dietary and lifestyle changes. In the end, however, the patients themselves create health (and then they are so kind that they earn their doctor an award!).

A Program for Life

The Maximum Healing Diet and Lifestyle Program is composed of four parts. I recommend that you give yourself a week to fully incorporate each aspect of the program into your life before adding the next. Of course, you are free to adopt the entire Maximum Healing Program at once, or to take longer to incorporate each aspect of the program into your life, if necessary.

Of the four parts, the first two weeks (or the first two aspects of the program)—the diet and exercise components—are the most important. I have found that if people change their eating habits and start exercising, the rest of their lives change for the better. They tend to take much better care of themselves, deal with stress more appropriately, and are more likely to live more balanced lives. For this reason, I maintain that people who really want to improve their lives begin with a healthier diet and a regular exercise program. No matter what else you do, those two steps are essential.

In addition to diet and exercise programs, I provide recommendations for reducing stress and achieving a more balanced existence in weeks three and four. Throughout this book, I report many of the dramatic results people have had with the Maximum Healing Program. People who were given little chance of improving were able to restore their health entirely and wean themselves off all medications. I am confident that if you adopt this program, you will see remarkable improvement in your own life, as well.

I have provided two diets in Chapter Ten. Both are, in fact, Liv-its, but I will use the word "diet" because that is what people are mostly used to. The diet you choose to follow will depend on your current health status and how significant you want your results to be.

The first diet is called the Good Health Maintenance Diet. The second is the Maximum Healing Diet.

The Good Health Maintenance diet is intended for those who are in relatively good health and not severely overweight. These people want to increase energy; lose some weight; boost their immune and cancer-fighting systems; eliminate mild, chronic symptoms; and prevent disease.

Those who adopt the Maximum Healing Diet want to lose weight healthfully and quickly and overcome existing disorders, such as heart disease, type 2 diabetes, obesity, allergies, asthma, and other immune-related problems. Among the benefits you can experience by following the Maximum Healing Diet:

- The significant improvement or elimination of symptoms from major illnesses, including chest pain, adult-onset (type 2) diabetes, peripheral arterial disease (PAD) and its associated troubles such as claudication (the cramp-like calf pains experienced by patients with poor circulation in their legs), and high blood pressure
- A marked increase in energy and endurance
- Significant weight loss
- Prevention and/or amelioration of serious illnesses, including heart disease, cancer, high blood pressure, and adult-onset diabetes as a consequence of the dramatic improvement in immune and cancer-fighting systems
- Balanced hormones and the reduction in the risk of breast, ovarian, uterine, and prostate cancers

- A sharp reduction in or elimination of allergy symptoms
- Significant improvement or elimination of joint pain from rheumatoid arthritis
- Significant reduction in blood cholesterol and triglycerides
- Greater mental clarity, sharper thinking, and improved memory
- More healthy and youthful skin and overall appearance
- Heightened sense of well-being, reduction in stress, and a more positive and hopeful outlook on life

The Maximum Healing Diet and Lifestyle can also be used as an adjunct treatment for a wide variety of illnesses, including cancer. (See Chapter Six for more on the use of the Maximum Healing Diet and Lifestyle for the treatment of cancer.)

In Chapter Seven, I provide a supplement and herbal program designed to address the following systems and conditions:

- Arthritis pain and other symptoms
- Asthma, allergies, nasal congestion, and colds
- Bone density and strength
- Digestion
- Emotions and related disorders, including anxiety and depression
- Clarity of mind and memory
- Headaches and migraines
- Heart disease and high cholesterol
- Immune and cancer-fighting systems
- Prostate disorders

I use this program to treat people in my practice every day of the week. The results are often startling, as so many of my patients have discovered. Let's turn now to examine more carefully how the immune system works, and how you can make it stronger to regain your own health.

CHAPTER TWO

Experiencing Your Immune System

Twenty-eight-year-old Elaine had recently immigrated to the United States from Jamaica. She was 115 pounds overweight and had a chronically depressed immune system. "If some germ is in the air, doctor, I find a way to catch it," she used to say to me in her beautiful Jamaican accent. She had been taking over-the-counter medications that were costing her a small fortune, as well as periodic antibiotics to treat bacterial infections. She had chronic constipation and indigestion—thanks in part to the antibiotics that were killing her friendly intestinal bacteria. In one of our discussions, she admitted that she overate because she always found herself in relationships with men that were unsatisfying and sometimes downright abusive.

"Elaine, you've got to make a big change in your life," I told her one day. "And that change has to begin with your health. If you don't lose weight, you're going to have a heart attack or get some form of cancer— maybe colon cancer, maybe breast cancer. I promise you that if you change your way of eating and you exercise regularly, you will see a lot of other problems in your life clear up."

"I know," she told me. "I'm going to get really sick if I don't do something."

"Okay," I said. "Here's what you do."

I gave her my dietary and exercise program. I took her off of all red meat, chicken, and dairy products—she could have soy and rice milk, but no cheese or cow's milk. I wanted her to eat two servings a day of cooked whole grains, especially brown rice, barley, and millet. I also wanted her to eat between five and seven servings of vegetables per day, along with one or two pieces of fruit.

In the beginning, she could eat as much fish as she liked. I wanted her to eat vegetable soup every day. There are many healthful vegetable soup products available in cans, or in dehydrated form, which can be heated in minutes. She could also eat rice cakes and add rice syrup as a sweetener, or add natural jams and spreads to rice cakes. As much as possible, I wanted her to avoid bread and other processed foods. I gave her an antioxidant formula and a probiotic supplement that would help repopulate her intestines and promote better elimination. (See Chapter Eight for more on supplements.)

Over the next fifteen months, Elaine ate an incredibly healthy diet and exercised four times a week. Her exercise achieved the two cardinal rules of success and health: exercise to a sweat and shortness of breath simultaneously. In a little more than a year, she lost 112 pounds.

Her intestinal health and immune strength improved remarkably. Elaine had a very strong constitution to begin with and now her abundant energy reserves and natural strength could be used for more than just carrying an extra hundred pounds around. Needless to say, she no longer caught every cold and flu that turned up in the environment. But in addition to all of that, Elaine also went through a personal and physical transformation of the type that restores one's belief in the inherent strength and wisdom of people.

As she lost weight, her self-esteem improved dramatically. Eventually, she got rid of two boyfriends in succession—"Neither of them was worth keeping," she told me one day—and she got a better job. When she started to lose significant amounts of weight, she began to realize that buried below all those excess pounds was a beautiful, talented woman who deserved the very best life could give her. Now she felt ready to receive more from life.

Elaine is an example of the kind of rebirth people can experience when they eat a healthy diet and exercise regularly. Indeed, the human body possesses miraculous restorative powers. No system better illustrates those powers than our immune systems.

What Marvels the Immune System Performs!

The immune system's job is to recognize disease-causing agents in your system such as bacteria, viruses, fungi, or cancer cells, and to create a response that is capable of destroying that threat to your health. The immune system does this by being able to distinguish "self" from "not self." This means it can recognize your cells, proteins, and chemical factors and tell them apart from foreign substances that have invaded your system.

On the surface, that sounds pretty impressive, and indeed it is, but when you look closer at the system's sensory abilities, you cannot help but be astounded. Allow me to explain. Let's say that your immune system looks at two different proteins, each of which is composed of hundreds of amino acids, the building blocks of proteins. And let's say that the only difference between these two proteins is a single amino acid, or one building block out of several hundred. Your immune system can not only tell the difference between the two proteins, but can also determine which one is you, and whether or not the other is a threat to your health. In fact, your defenses can recognize literally millions of different disease-causing agents—otherwise known as antigens—and come up with a highly creative and highly effective response to each one.

As if all of that weren't impressive enough, the immune system accomplishes yet another remarkable feat: it remembers everything—what the antigen looked like and exactly which immune formula was created to destroy it. That's why you rarely, if ever, suffer from the same cold or flu virus more than once. All your immune system needs is a single exposure to a bacteria or virus to know just what to do about it for the rest of your life.

On top of all of that, the system shuts itself down when it sees that the threat to your health has been eliminated. If it didn't turn itself off, it would destroy you.

Every day, your immune system goes through this cycle of recognition, response, and shutdown—and all the while, you are oblivious to such miraculous activity.

The immune system is also categorized by the nature of its components: cellular and humoral, which is composed of antibodies, proteins, and chemical messengers. It is also divided into two main categories: innate immunity and acquired immunity.

Innate characteristics are those you were born with; the acquired abilities are those that you have developed by living in a disease-infested world.

Acquired immunity is a direct outgrowth of the system's capacity to experience diseases and remember what to do about each one.

As I mentioned earlier, the immune system is an army—an army whose numbers are inconceivable. In its relaxed state, the system is composed of roughly a *trillion* cells; that's a million million! To put that number in another way, think of it as a million groups of cells, with each group having a million members. As I said, it's inconceivable. As long as there are sufficient immune boosters on reserve (more about immune boosters in the next chapter), their numbers will continue to multiply.

A brief look at a few of the basic elements of your immune defenses will give you an idea of just how creative, powerful, and even miraculous this system really is.

Basic Elements of Your Immune System

Complement: Poking Holes in the Enemy's Defenses

Complement is a group of proteins that circulate in the blood. Once the complement protein perceives an antagonist (pathogen), it attempts to destroy it by poking holes in its cell membrane, thus causing its death. Complement also has the tendency to poke holes in nearby blood vessels, causing blood and fluid to leak into tissues. That action stimulates the arrival of other immune cells—rather like sending up a flare for help.

The Granulocytes and Monocytes: The First Line of Defense

Granulocytes and monocytes are the white blood cells, which create pus, that unlovely word we use to describe the white yellow fluid that gathers in infected cuts. Granulocytes and monocytes show up at the places where we are bruised, cut, or physically injured, the very places where bacteria and viruses try to enter our system and create problems.

Once on the scene, these cells start ingesting bacteria and viruses. Once ingested, the invaders are plunged into the granulocytes' and monocytes' stomachs, or lysosomes, where there are such highly toxic fluids as hydrogen peroxide, nitric oxide, and hypochlorite (the active ingredient in bleach), which destroy those invading organisms. Granulocytes and monocytes are also known as phagocytes, a term that means, "to ingest and digest microorganisms."

One drawback: granulocytes can produce an excess of these powerful chemical substances, and then these toxic substances can be released into healthy tissues. Once released, these chemicals produce oxidants and inflammation. Eventually, they can also kill healthy cells. For this reason, scientists describe granulocytes as imprecise, even sloppy. Like a shotgun, they're effective, but they can leave a mess behind.

The Macrophage: Smart, Deadly, and Blessed with Powerful Friends

Macrophages, which are far more sophisticated and powerful immune cells than granulocytes and monocytes, are like blind people with very sensitive fingers. These cells have "fingers" named "toll-like receptors" (TLRs) ("toll" is the German word for "weird" or "far-out"—*Science* 2006; 312:184-187). Like a blind person who identifies objects and even people by touch, macrophages recognize the identity of an antigen by bumping up against it and feeling its physical body with sensitive, antennae-like projections that radiate from the macrophage's cell wall.

Once it frisks the unknown intruder, the macrophage sends the information it has gleaned back to its nucleus, which processes it, and identifies the bad guy. "Yikes! Streptococcus bacteria," the macrophage might say to itself. Unless you are an infant, the chances are very good that you have encountered strep many times before. The nucleus of the macrophage informs the cell of just what it needs to do to destroy the strep, long before it can do any damage. Just as the granulocytes had done, the macrophages can produce an array of highly toxic chemicals to kill the invader, including hydrogen peroxide, nitric oxide, and hypochlorite.

Like granulocytes, macrophages can phagocytize, or gobble up, bacteria and viruses, but they can also call on other immune cells, thus triggering a far more elaborate and powerful reaction from the immune system.

Let's say that a particular macrophage cell was the first to bump into strep bacteria. Chances are good that strep is in other places within the system. In order to alert the rest of the system to the presence of strep, the macrophage will release an array of chemical messengers, called cytokines (chemical messages that are "cell movers"), which not only trigger a body-wide immune response, but may also induce sleep. If the strep poses a sufficient threat, the macrophages might release other cytokines that would produce fever and the full-blown symptoms of a cold ("strep" or "sore throat," for example). As I explained in the last chapter, many of these cold symptoms are the immune system's way of coping with the bacteria or virus.

Macrophages also encounter, identify, and kill cancer cells. Whenever that happens, macrophages produce another cytokine, called tumor necrosis factor, a chemical capable of destroying cancer cells and tumors. Again, too much of that can be a problem.

Finally, if the macrophages recognize that the antigen is too powerful for them alone, they call out the immune system's four-star generals, the T-lymphocytes, otherwise known as T-helper CD4 cells. The CD4 T-helper cells are the brains of the operation. They alone are capable of bringing to bear all of the immune system's incredible forces to the fight against a disease. When the CD4 cells enter the struggle, the battle of the cells against the antigen heats up significantly.

Lymphocytes: Intelligence, Power, and Command

The most powerful immune cells in your system only enter the battlefield when called upon to act. And the only way they are brought into the battle is when the macrophages make them realize that their help is needed. Remarkably, it's not as simple a step as you might think. The macrophages have to coax the CD4 cells into action.

The way in which the macrophages do this suggests not only respect for the CD4 cell, but reverence. When macrophages encounter an invader and recognize that greater help is needed, they gobble up the antigen and then regurgitate bits of the invader's proteins. Those small pieces of protein are then placed in cup-like structures that extend from the macrophages' cell membranes. These structures are called major histocompatibility complexes (MHCs). The macrophages, in effect, are offering up these tiny bits of protein, hoping that the CD4 cells recognize them as a bonafide threat to the system. In a kind of massive candlelight vigil, millions of macrophages do this at once.

Recognition is not a *fait accompli,* unfortunately. A CD4 cell can only respond to the presence of an antigen if, and only if, it has the right kind of receptor that responds to that specific kind of illness. The receptor emanates from the CD4's cell membrane and resembles a whip-like antenna. Although CD4 cells have many antennae emanating from their surfaces, each cell has only one type of receptor, which means that each CD4 T-helper cell can only recognize one type of illness. It's rather like having lots of telephone lines coming into a home, but each can receive calls from only one particular person. Each CD4 cell is capable of receiving calls only from one specific type of illness.

That is not to say that there is only one CD4 cell for each illness. Actually, there are whole families of CD4 cells that have the same type of receptor. But each family can identify and react to only one disease.

Let's say that there's a streptococcus bacteria afoot in your system. Circulating in your bloodstream and lurking in your tissues is a big family of CD4 cells that have the receptors for streptococcus. But there are millions and millions more CD4 cells that do not have that receptor, and therefore do not respond to strep when they see it. That means that millions of CD4 cells are simply passing by all of those macrophage cells that are offering up tiny bits of strep for recognition.

Macrophages offer up those little bits of protein until a CD4 cell with the right receptor happens along and recognizes the antigen's protein. Fortunately for all of us, that event eventually occurs. And when that happens, the entire immune system is suddenly switched on. It's as if electrical power were suddenly restored to New York City in the middle of the night.

The first thing that the CD4 cell does when it recognizes an illness is to replicate itself over and over again. Those CD4 T-helper cells that have the right receptor for this illness are now multiplying rapidly. Hordes of them are traveling throughout your body via the bloodstream. In effect, the right generals are taking their positions throughout the battlefield—in your sinuses, throat, liver, spleen, digestive tract, pelvis, legs, and toes.

The command centers are established. Next, a communications network is set up. That means that your system is now flooded with cytokines. Among the powerful immune cells called into battle are the natural killer

(NK) cells. Like highly trained soldiers, they attack viruses and/or cancer cells and tumors. These cells are highly effective, as long as they can identify the enemy and have the right environment to work within. By that I mean they need an environment that is itself not overly toxic, nor depleted in immune-boosting nutrients. The toxicity of the biological environment and the reserves of nutrients within that environment are dependent, of course, on our behaviors. But given the right conditions, the army of immune cells is capable of wiping out just about anything.

In fact, the CD4 cells can make all of the immune constituents even more effective, thanks to their ability to produce cytokines.

Cytokines: Rounding Up and Inspiring the Troops

Among the most important cytokines (cell movers) that are produced are the interleukins, designated IL-1 through IL-33. These are powerfully charged catalysts that have specialized effects on the immune system. IL-2, for example, stimulates the whole army of immune cells to divide and replicate. Other interleukins produce all the symptoms that we normally associate with sickness—inflammation, increased heat in the tissues, increased blood flow throughout the system, fever, aches and pains, grumpiness, sleepiness, and fatigue.

Still others stimulate macrophages and lymphocytes to produce tumor necrosis factor. A group of interleukins triggers the production of gamma-interferon, which interferes with the genes of viruses, thus preventing them from reproducing themselves. Another form of interferon is also produced, which ignites the passions of the natural killer cells, making them all the more rabid and destructive.

Interleukins 2, 4, and 6 cause T lymphocytes, macrophages, and natural killer cells to become cytotoxic cells—that is, to become cell-killers, or immune cells that destroy cancer cells and cells that have been taken over by viruses.

Certain interleukins cause complement, macrophages, and natural killer cells to become more aggressive in the face of a disease, ravenously gobbling up cancer cells, viruses, or bacteria.

At this point in the battle, wonders beyond anything the human imagination could conceive are taking place. Genes are being shuffled to produce chemical antidotes to illnesses. A trial-and-error process is occurring as cells experiment with each chemical antidote, analyze its effectiveness, and decide whether to keep using it or go for a better approach.

Behind all these explosive events, the CD4 cells continue to orchestrate the immune response. Having brought in all kinds of fighting forces, which have been catalyzed to a fever pitch, the CD4 cells call in yet another set of soldiers, the B cells, or what might otherwise be called the magicians.

Antibodies: Brilliant Destructive Powers and No Small Humor

B cells are not the rabid killers that granulocytes, monocytes, natural killer cells, and even macrophages are. They're more cerebral than physically destructive. Yet they are incredibly effective. Their mission is to produce antibodies, also known as immunoglobulins, which are the chemical antidotes to disease.

B cells arrive on the scene and immediately assess what they are up against. Then they start juggling and activating genes to produce any number of highly creative responses to disease. Among B cells favorite responses are the following:

- They can produce highly toxic chemicals that can destroy viruses, bacteria, and cancer cells.
- They can produce chemicals that are used to coat a pathogen. Some of those chemicals attract natural killer cells, macrophages, granulocytes, and monocytes to the pathogens. Others attract complement. The strategy is rather like draping a bad guy in meat and then releasing the lions.
- They also produce a substance that acts like glue, which they use to cover the virus or bacteria. The glue causes the disease-causing cells to stick together and become even more visible to the immune system. In other words, they stick out like a band of gangsters in church.
- Another strategy is to produce a chemical substance that makes viruses, bacteria, and cancer cells exceedingly slippery, as if they've been bathed in oil, thus preventing these disease-causing agents from gaining a foothold in the system.

As the immune system is fighting the battle, it's also taking notes, so to speak. It remembers everything that worked, filing this information away to be retrieved and activated the minute the same bad-guy shows up again in the system.

Once the battle has been won, the system recognizes its victory and shuts itself down. It does this by stimulating production of CD8 suppressor cells, whose responsibility is to gradually wind down and turn off the system. Were it not for these cells, the immune system would become a monster and destroy you in no time flat.

It is the unhealthy ratio of CD4 to CD8 cells that characterizes the perilous situation people with AIDS find themselves in. As the disease progresses, CD4 cells die off, causing CD8 cells to far outnumber their brethren. With CD8 cells in the majority, the system keeps shutting itself off, even in the face of a disease that would otherwise stimulate a powerful immune response. As we will see in later chapters, there are ways to stimulate production of CD4 cells, and thus support the immune system's powers.

For most of us, however, the system remains largely in balance. It doesn't attack healthy tissues, nor does it shut down prematurely in the face of a pathogen. It is entirely benign, a giant whose sole purpose is to keep you alive.

The primary problem the immune system faces is whether or not there are adequate resources to keep it functioning at peak efficiency and strength. Unfortunately for most of us, our contemporary biological environment suppresses the health and strength of our immune systems. In addition, most of us do not provide the system with all it needs to function optimally. Let's look now at how our inner environments can affect our immune defenses.

A Healthy Response Sometimes Feels Like Sickness

In a strange and ironic sort of way, the immune system gives rise to symptoms that most of us think of as sickness. The symptoms that you may regard as illness—a fever, for example, or inflammation—are actually tools used by the immune system to rid your body of illness. Here are a few examples:

- Fever. Macrophages release cytokines that elevate the body's temperature and create fever. Scientists believe that the immune system creates fever in order to make the conditions within the system more hostile to the invading virus or pathogen.

- Inflammation. Immune cells often destroy pathogens by releasing oxidants, or highly reactive oxygen molecules that cause the breakdown and death of viruses and bacteria. Granulocytes, monocytes, and macrophages attack bacteria and viruses literally by eating them. Once the pathogen is inside the immune cell's stomach, it is destroyed by powerful digestive juices that include hydrogen peroxide, nitric oxide, and hypochlorite (as said before, the active ingredient in bleach). These substances all release free radicals, which in turn produce inflammation. Macrophages also release oxidants as powerful weapons against disease, and such oxidants also produce inflammation.

- Inflammation is also caused by interleukins (IL-1 all the way through IL-33). Interleukins trigger a more powerful immune reaction by causing immune cells to reproduce rapidly in face of a threat to health. They also produce inflammation, which increases heat and blood circulation in the area. That, in turn, attracts a stronger immune response.

- Finally, inflammation is also caused by the release of histamine, a chemical produced by mast cells, which arrive on the scene whenever there is an injury. By creating inflammation, mast cells ensure that more immune cells will be attracted to an area.

- Of course, when a great crowd of immune cells and chemical factors arrive on the scene, inevitably there is an even greater production of oxidants, which often increase inflammation, as well.

- Fatigue and sleepiness. The immune system is a marvel of efficiency. When it confronts a threat to your health, it mobilizes as much energy as the body can divert to combating the illness. Thus, one of the steps the immune system takes is to shut down all unnecessary activity. Macrophages and their cytokines—especially IL-1 and interferon—accomplish this by creating deep fatigue and sleepiness. Once you are immobilized, so to speak, your immune system can utilize the energy you would otherwise use for working on more important matters—namely overcoming the pathogen or disorder and restoring your health.

- Red coloring, especially around a sore, cut, or bruise, is often caused when complement releases a chemical that causes blood vessels to leak. This alerts the immune system to send out more cells to a particular part of the body.
- Cough. Coughing is a reflex action caused by the presence of inflammation—usually the consequence of an immune reaction—in the lungs, bronchial tubes, and throat. Coughing is also triggered by the presence of an irritating agent, such as mucous, smoke, or toxic chemicals, in those areas.
- Irritability. That irritability, grumpiness, and sensitivity you feel when you get sick is no accident. Cytokines regulate hormones, including cortisol, to make you feel antisocial. This forces you to stop working, get plenty of rest, and avoid social contact. This latter step is especially designed to keep you from encountering people who might introduce another pathogen to your system.
- Joint pain, muscle ache, and headache. Interleukins 1 and 2 combine to produce inflammation, joint pain, muscle aches, and headache. Though scientists aren't sure why these effects occur, we do know that they get our attention fast by making work or play uncomfortable or virtually impossible. All we want to do is take to our beds, which is exactly the response your defenses need from you.

Whenever any of these symptoms occur, you should be aware that your immune system is fighting for your life. Long before you get ill—and especially before you are severely ill—you may experience one or several of these symptoms. Any sudden or chronic problem can serve as an early warning system, alerting you to the fact that your defenses are hard at work and need your support and attention. Among the most common early signals of illness are:

- Chronic fatigue, lasting weeks at a time, often associated with an increased demand for sleep
- Allergies or persistent allergic symptoms
- Chronic headaches
- Joint pain or another form of chronic pain
- A chronic skin irritation, or skin eruptions, such as from eczema or psoriasis
- A chronic cold, cough, or sinus infection that cannot be shaken
- Asthma attacks
- Imbalanced lifestyle, such as a disproportionate amount of time spent working, out of work, alone, or answering the demands of others
- The presence of a chronic illness that cannot be overcome

Fighting the System That Tries to Save Your Life

Unfortunately, those of us who live in the Western hemisphere have been taught to suppress the very activities that the immune system uses to restore health. All too often, we use over-the-counter or prescription medicines to suppress fever, reduce inflammation, stop mucous discharge, and artificially boost energy so that we can conduct our lives as usual.

Rather than resting and allowing the body to heal, we often use drugs to circumvent and undermine the healing process. While is may be true that some medicines weaken the causes of illness, research from the March 1993 issue of *Folia Bioligica* reported that some drugs, particularly antibiotics, do indeed weaken the immune system.

Drugs suppress the activities of the immune response and replace immune activities. One of the fundamental laws of the body is "If you don't use it, you lose it." This goes for muscle, bone, and mental functioning. It also appears to apply to the immune system.

Excessive use of drugs appear to weaken the overall immune response, which is exactly what we do not want to happen in an age when illnesses are becoming increasingly resistant to our most powerful pharmaceuticals. There is, however, a time and place for everything.

Interestingly, ancient or traditional forms of medicine, such as Greek, Chinese, and Ayurvedic (Hindu), recognized all of these symptoms as the body's attempt to rid itself of disease. Ancient healers regarded symptoms, such as those described above, as the body's method of healing itself. For example, for thousands of years Chinese medicine taught that a runny nose, sneezing, mucous discharge, cough, frequent urination, and diarrhea were all attempts by the body to rid itself of the sources of disease. Traditional healers, such as the Chinese, attempted to work with the body to help it cleanse itself of the sources of illness. This makes sense to me.

This was the case with Hippocrates, as well. Hippocrates, the Greek physician and father of medicine, taught that the symptoms of illness were, in fact, an orderly process undertaken by the body to reestablish health. Hippocrates maintained that the physician should intervene at just the right moment in the healing process—a moment he referred to as the *kairos,* or crisis. At this moment, the physician could apply his art to encourage the forces of healing, which Hippocrates called *pepsis,* and assist the body in overcoming the illness.

This is one of the many things modern medicine is learning from traditional healing systems: we must support the body in its own healing process, rather than try to substitute medication for the powerful immune system that is already in place. This is where immune boosters enter the picture.

Much of what we know about the immune system today we have learned during the last two decades, since the rise of HIV and AIDS. Although our knowledge of the immune system is relatively young, it is also growing quickly.

Among the most important lessons science is learning is that our immune defenses need our help on a daily basis. Diet, nutritional supplements, herbs, moderate exercise, and the types of thoughts and emotions that we engage in determine the strength of our defenses. Indeed, lifestyle may determine the quality of your health.

If you are experiencing robust good health, abundant energy, clarity of mind, and deep, restful sleep, your immune system is probably working optimally. Your body is not being weakened by any number of possible antagonists. Your energy is not being diverted to the job of overcoming some deeply entrenched disease. But if you feel stressed or anxious, or suffer from chronic illness, injury, physical complaint, or serious disease, then your immune system is probably under siege. In other words, it's time to take your natural defenses seriously and start supporting them.

CHAPTER THREE

How and Why This Program Works

Melanie, forty-nine, a postmenopausal businesswoman and the mother of two grown children, had suffered from allergies for twenty years. Melanie originally came to me for relief from an array of immune-related symptoms, including nasal allergies, watery eyes, chronic headaches, joint pain, and chronically low energy. She was about twenty-five pounds overweight, which, on her five-foot-five frame, was significant. During that first visit, I checked her blood pressure, did an electrocardiogram, and discovered that Melanie had mild hypertension with signs of heart disease. I asked Melanie if she was careful with her diet. "Oh yes," she told me. "I try to eat as healthy as I can."

Her response did not carry much weight with me. Many of my patients tell me, during our first visit, that they try to eat a healthful diet. It's only later, after we start working together, that they realize that my idea of a healthy diet is often very different from their own and dramatically different from The Maximum Healing Diet.

A series of blood tests found that Melanie's blood cholesterol level was 223 milligrams per deciliter with triglycerides at 380 milligrams per deciliter, both of which confirmed that she was in serious jeopardy of having a heart attack (average heart attack levels are 205 and 225 respectively).

Melanie also had low blood levels of magnesium, always a sign to me of a poor diet and predisposition to diabetes. Magnesium is concentrated in plant foods. Therefore, the most common reason for low magnesium levels is a diet rich in animal and processed foods and low in whole grains, fresh vegetables, and beans. Her high cholesterol and triglyceride levels and her excess weight supported that deduction. If one is dedicated to a grain-vegetable-beans (**GVB**) "Liv-it" with some nuts, seeds, fruits, and fish about twice a week, it is almost impossible to become overweight.

Blood cholesterol is elevated mostly by saturated fat, which is found in red meats, pork, eggs, and cheeses, but also by an elevated percentage of body fat. Triglycerides, another blood fat, increase as a consequence of too many calories, especially from sugar and processed foods, such as rolls, cakes, pastries, white bread, and soft drinks. In other words, Melanie was a junk-food eater.

I went over my standard four-week dietary plan with her. I carefully described the foods she should eat during each week. The desk in my office is covered with a wide variety of healthful foods that can be purchased in most grocery or natural foods stores. They include a variety of whole grains—such as brown rice, millet, oats, and barley—beans, vegetables, whole-grain noodles, soups, sauces, and quick meals, all vegetable-based and all designed to boost immunity and lower cholesterol and triglyceride levels. As I described each food, I handed her a small bag or can that contained the food I was talking about. I also gave her written instructions (my patient education handouts are available at www.thepmc.org) on how to prepare each of the items I described.

I work with several cooking teachers and nutritionists in the greater Hartford area who offer wonderful natural foods cooking classes.

"I'd like you to stop eating all forms of dairy food," I told Melanie. "Dairy may be causing your allergies. Cow's milk and milk products contain proteins that, in sensitive people, can stimulate an immune response that is experienced as an allergic reaction. Also, dairy food contains saturated fat, which is raising your cholesterol and triglyceride levels and affecting your heart. Please stop the dairy foods, and let's see what happens."

I gave her a list of dairy substitutes—rice and soymilk, along with soymilk cheeses—and showed her such products.

I then recommended a combination of food-based supplements that included antioxidants, especially vitamins C, E (an E with all eight components), and mixed carotenoids, probiotics, and digestive enzymes. (See Chapters Eight and Twelve for more on supplements and diet, respectively.)

I also recommended a variety of immune-boosting behaviors, including a daily walk. "You don't need to power walk, Melanie," I said. "Just walk for half an hour a day. If you can't get a thirty-minute walk in, then take one or two ten-minute walks to start. Even that small amount of exercise will have a tremendous impact on your health."

"Finally," I said, "I'd like you to stop drinking coffee every day. Getting rid of coffee will reduce, and possibly even eliminate your tension and headaches. Drink green or black tea, such as English Breakfast, and make it progressively weaker over time until you are no longer dependent on caffeine." I have found that a cup of English Breakfast tea, made with two tea bags instead of one, provides enough of a boost to substitute for one cup of coffee.

Within the next three months, Melanie had made remarkable progress. She lost twenty pounds and got into an exercise routine. She had done splendidly on the Liv-it (diet) I recommended. Both of those factors eliminated her hypertension. Her cholesterol level fell to 180 milligrams per deciliter—not perfect, but more acceptable to me. (I prefer the cholesterol level to be at 150 milligrams per deciliter or less and that "non-HDL" cholesterol be less than ninety milligrams per deciliter. Please see the complete list of Wellness Protection and Disease Prevention Goals in the Appendix.) Her triglycerides fell to a perfect sixty milligrams per deciliter. The reductions in cholesterol and triglycerides indicated that she had dramatically reduced her saturated fat intake, total calories, and processed foods. She was no longer eating as many animal foods, fast foods and "white" foods. As far as I was concerned, she was making great progress and out of immediate danger of having a heart attack.

Her allergies cleared up, as did her joint pain, headaches, and chronic fatigue. She told me that she felt better than she had since she was in her twenties.

How to Boost Immunity

Immune boosting is the foundation of The Maximum Healing Program, which really means restoring your health. Maximum Healing depends on two factors: cleanup and immune boosting.

Cleanup means reducing as much as possible the poisons that are polluting your internal biochemistry. These toxins cause all the big, life-threatening illnesses: heart disease, cancer, high blood pressure, and adult-onset diabetes. Toxins also create an internal environment that's more susceptible to viral and bacterial infection.

As you reduce the toxic burden in your body, your immune system can direct more of its energy and attention to the actual diseases from which you may be suffering. But there's more to it than that. Certain substances that we consume—especially excesses of anything, but specifically excess dietary fat, processed carbohydrates, and sugars—disrupt communication between, and within, immune cells. This causes individual cells to malfunction and the overall immune response to be weaker.

The second set of behaviors is, strictly speaking, immune boosting. Immune-boosting behaviors increase the number and aggressiveness of immune cells. They also promote greater production of cytokines, the chemical messengers, and tumor necrosis factor, a powerful cancer fighter.

Among the immune boosters are many nutrients, plant chemicals, and physical behaviors such as moderate exercise, meditation, prayer, and stress reduction. As you will see, your social life plays a role in the relative health of your immune system, as well.

Cleaning up your biochemical environment and engaging in immune-strengthening behaviors can be seen as the yin and yang of immune boosting. Neither side works as well without the other. You need to do both to get your system to run at peak performance.

In this chapter, we'll consider the big picture of how certain everyday actions can dramatically improve your health.

The First Great Burden to Your Immune System: Oxidants

Oxidants (not to be confused with the biologically friendly antioxidants) are types of oxygen molecules that interact with neighboring molecules and cause them to decay. They do that by causing their neighbors to lose electrons. A molecule has the same number of electrons as protons; when an electron is lost; the molecule becomes unstable and starts to break down neighboring molecules to get that electron back. These molecules, in turn, steal electrons from their neighbors. An unstable molecule that causes the breakdown of a neighboring molecule is called a free radical.

When a whole neighborhood of molecules starts stealing electrons from each other, you've got pure chaos. Cells and tissues break down and become deformed. Cells die. Tissue shrinks and forms scar tissue. When this process occurs in the brain, it forms the basis for Alzheimer's and Parkinson's disease. When it occurs in the eyes, it turns clear lenses into opaque clouds (cataracts). When it occurs in the liver, kidneys, or other major organs, it causes them to shrivel up and lose their functional capacity. When it occurs in the coronary arteries (the vessels that bring blood to the heart), it forms cholesterol plaques, or boils, within the artery walls. Eventually those plaques can rupture and form a clot that can become large enough to block blood flow to the heart and cause a heart attack. When oxidants cause changes in the DNA of cells, many cells die, but some can start reproducing uncontrollably. They can become malignant forms of cancer.

Longtime cancer researcher, Bruce Ames, PhD, director of Biochemical Research at the University of California at Berkeley, has determined that human DNA is assaulted by ten thousand oxidant hits per day. That assault is a constant barrage of oxidants. Fortunately, every cell is equipped with enzymes and antioxidants that immediately repair damage to DNA. But it's up to us to keep replenishing those antioxidant levels. Otherwise, the effects of that daily bombardment could be fatal.

Oxidants are likely the primary cause behind more than sixty major illnesses. They also underlie the process by which aging occurs. Aging is really the rate at which your cells and tissues decay. To a great extent, you control the speed with which your tissues break down, shrink, and become deformed, by controlling the amount of oxidation that takes place in your tissues.

Oxidants are caused by an array of environmental factors, including tobacco smoking, dietary fat, cholesterol, alcohol consumption, processed foods, and pesticides in food, excess sunlight, sedentary lifestyle, and chemical pollutants in the air, water, and soil.

The thoughts you think and the emotional life that you experience every day can also alter your hormonal environment and raise the oxidant level in our tissues. If you don't get enough sleep, or are unable to enjoy deep sleep, your immune system will not be as effective at warding off disease. Also, your body will not be able to repair cells as effectively.

The five factors that I outlined in Chapter One—air, water, food, level of physical activity, and the kinds emotions and thoughts you experience—all play major roles in determining how rapidly you age.

You cannot avoid oxidation entirely, because it occurs as a normal part of cellular metabolism and immune activity. Immune cells use oxidants to destroy bacteria and viruses. The body has many built-in mechanisms for protecting itself against these sources of oxidants, including its own antioxidant reserves and protective mechanisms that protect cells and DNA.

Also, your immune system recognizes oxidants and free radicals as a threat to your health. Immune cells scavenge, or gobble up, oxidants and free radicals, thus preventing them from doing harm to your body. But the more oxidants in your system, the more your immune system is constantly engaged in the struggle to eliminate them.

Oxidants are like small, out-of-control fires taking place in your tissues. Your immune system is like your own inner fire department. If the fire department constantly has to deal with small fires raging throughout the system, it never has the time, energy, or resources to deal with the really dangerous fires that are occurring elsewhere.

Your lifestyle, especially your diet, can add significantly to your oxidative load. Your lifestyle and diet can increase oxidants levels so far that they overcome your built-in protective mechanisms. That's when things become dangerous. At that point, your risk of illness goes up exponentially.

All of us have some susceptibility to one or another degenerative disease. One may have susceptibility or a genetic predisposition, (that is you are genetically programmed to have a predisposition) for cancer, another for heart disease, and still another for adult-onset diabetes. Many people have a greater than average susceptibility (genetic predisposition) for Alzheimer's or Parkinson's.

When the oxidant load overrides antioxidant capacities, those genes that would give rise to one or another of these diseases are more likely to express themselves and you may fall prey to the disease to which you are predisposed. In other words, oxidants create an environment in which genes for a specific kind of illness are more likely to be expressed and then give rise to that disease.

However, just because you have a particular predisposed weakness for heart disease or cancer does not mean that you are destined to get either of those diseases. On the contrary, environmental conditions may determine whether your genes will trigger that disease. Perhaps the most important factor needed to create that sickness-producing environment is the excess production of oxidants. Limiting your oxidant burden is the first step toward greater health.

This is why antioxidants are so important. They slow down and even stop the oxidative process. They do it by donating electrons to imbalanced molecules, thus providing molecules with their requisite number of electrons and stabilize them. This essentially brings peace and stability to the neighborhood, as Mr. Rogers might say.

Antioxidants also protect DNA from attack by free radicals. They are part of the system built into every cell that restores health and stability to the cell's brain center.

The Big Sources of Oxidants (Oxidation)

Protecting the body, and specifically the immune system, from the damaging effects of oxidants means limiting their sources. To protect yourself from oxidants, stay away from cigarette smoking, excess exposure to sunlight, alcohol, and dietary fat. In other words, protect your body from unhealthy air, water, and diet. Once you have taken care of these four, you can more easily control—and tolerate—some of the other sources. At the same time, you must build up your antioxidants and other immune-boosting reserves.

Dr. Ames, the Director of Biochemical Research at the University of California, Berkeley, has established that there are more than a million oxidants in a single puff of cigarette smoke. People who smoke age more rapidly than those who do not. They also have far greater risk of heart disease, cancer, and various disorders of the lungs and airways.

Women who smoke have a higher risk of osteoporosis and more wrinkled skin. There is no way that you can counteract the effects of smoking by taking supplements or eating a good diet. Cigarette smoking is among the greatest producers of oxidants that humans are exposed to.

Unfortunately, you can inhale cigarette smoke without being a smoker. If you socialize in bars or work in an environment where people are allowed to smoke, you may be the victim of secondhand smoke. My advice is simple: try to avoid smoky environments and change the conditions where you work—make the workplace a smoke-free environment—or change jobs entirely. Obviously, your health is far more valuable than your job. When people try to argue that point, I tell them that, no matter what kind of job you hold, it's a lot easier to get another job than it is to get another pair of lungs or another heart. Get away from cigarette smoke. There is no greater source of air pollution for the vast majority of Americans.

Skin cancer rates are skyrocketing today, and the primary cause is excessive exposure to ultraviolet rays, either from natural sunlight or artificial tanning beds. The sun's ultraviolet rays break down molecules, set free radicals in motion, and deform cells and tissues. People who are chronically exposed to excessive sunlight age far more rapidly than those who avoid over-exposure.

Sun-worshippers suffer the consequences of highly wrinkled and leathery skin. They dry up early in life and look decades older than their actual years. Wear sunscreen when you go out. Titanium suncreens by Vanicream, Lavera, Jason, and Anthelios SX provide great protection from the sun. Look for a sunscreen with SPF 30 or higher, UVA protection, and three stars for UVB protection. Choose make-up and moisturizers that contain sunscreen. Wear light protective clothing and a hat while you're in the sun. When you go to the beach, sit under an umbrella between eleven o'clock in the morning and two o'clock in the afternoon. Enjoy the air, the water, and the warmth of the sun, but don't spend more than thirty minutes under its direct rays. And, by the way, twenty minutes of direct sun gives you all the vitamin D you need in one day, any more is not helpful. Two to three times a week is perfect.

Alcohol is another major producer of oxidants. It is toxic to the liver, heart, bone marrow, and muscles in any dose. In the liver, alcohol transforms healthy cells into hardened scar tissue that can cause cirrhosis. Alcohol is essentially a highly processed sugar that is transformed in the body to fat. An early stage of liver disease, often caused by excess alcohol consumption, is a condition called "fatty liver."

Fat, as you know, is a reserve source of fuel. In order to be utilized as fuel, fat cells easily break down and release fat molecules into the bloodstream. Unfortunately, that same characteristic makes fatty tissues the most susceptible to oxidation. Since alcohol is a big producer of fat, and is, at the same time, a producer of oxidants, it has a doubly toxic effect on your body, especially the liver.

Interestingly, vitamin E (with all four tocopherols and four tocotrienols) and coenzyme Q10 are especially effective at slowing the oxidative process of fatty tissues and stabilizing fat cells.

The liver is highly susceptible to oxidative stress, in part because so much oxidation naturally takes place within the liver. The liver is constantly transforming highly poisonous substances, including alcohol, into water-soluble compounds that are easily expelled from the body. Many of these toxic chemicals, including pesticides and other environmental poisons, are themselves oxidant producers. Like cigarette smoke, excess alcohol consumption also creates wrinkling of skin. The alcohol stimulates the collagen fibers below the surface of the skin to break down and shrivel up. What people do not realize is that alcohol is doing the same thing to their organs, including their liver, pancreas, and lungs.

Unlike cigarette smoke, some sources of alcohol, such as beer and wine, also contain antioxidants. For this reason, many people think that these are healthy drinks. However, the amount of antioxidants in beer and wine do not offset the effects of the alcohol, especially when it is consumed in excess.

I do not urge people to swear off alcohol entirely. I say party a little; four drinks or less per week are usually fine and well tolerated by the body, depending, of course, on the health of the individual. Hazardous alcohol intake starts at ten drinks a week or more than four drinks at one sitting for men. In women, problem alcohol intake starts at five drinks per week or three in one sitting.

The last of the big four oxidant producers is dietary fat. Fat not only results in great quantities of oxidants, but also has other damaging effects on the immune system.

Dietary Fat: Gumming Up the Works

There are few things more harmful to your immune system than excess consumption of dietary fat, which has the ability to gum up the works in more ways than one.

I mentioned earlier that macrophages and other immune cells, most notably CD4 cells, discern friend from foe by bumping into a given cell, bacteria, or virus. Once it lays its sensitive antennae on the surface of the object in question, it can determine its nature. That job requires a very sensitive antenna and cell membrane.

Fat can infiltrate the cell membrane, reducing its sensitivity and blocking the signals that flow from the antennae to the cell's nucleus. In effect, the macrophage or CD4 cell can no longer tell what it's encountering, which enables bacteria, virus, or cancer cells to proliferate. Fat blinds the immune system and keeps it from reacting in the face of a disease-causing agent.

That's not all it does, however. Having infiltrated the cell membrane, the fat then oxidizes, deforming the membrane and the immune cell itself. The flow of information to the nucleus is hampered considerably. The affected cell may respond only partially to a bacteria or virus. It may release only small amounts of cytokines or none at all. It may no longer be able to produce tumor necrosis factor in the face of a cancer cell.

B cells that have been deformed in this way may have only limited ability to produce antibodies. Research has shown that excess consumption of fish oils—which are polyunsaturated fats—decreases production of IL-1, IL-2, and IL-6. Among other things, these interleukins should stimulate immune cells to reproduce when confronted with an antigen. When these cytokines are reduced, the immune system does not react with the aggressiveness that it would otherwise possess.

Other studies have shown that excess consumption of omega-6 polyunsaturated fats depresses immune function, while they promote tumor growth. Omega-6 fats are derived from corn oil, safflower oil, sunflower oil, and many seed and nut oils. Omega-6s are especially common in processed foods and store-bought pastries, especially in those that contain partially hydrogenated vegetable oils. Foods that contains such oils, and there is a plethora of them, can be immune depressing and cancer promoting.

Interestingly, not all fats weaken the immune system. Omega-3 polyunsaturated fats—such as those found in cold-water fish including salmon, cod, flounder, sardines, mackerel, and haddock, as well as in sea algae, wild plants, pumpkin seeds, walnuts, and almonds—are immune boosting if not consumed to excess. They also strengthen the body's cancer-fighting mechanisms. Research has shown that omega-3s make the cancer cells more vulnerable to chemotherapy and radiation but remarkably, omega-3s do not weaken the normal cells or make them more susceptible to cell death from chemotherapy and radiation. Using omega-3s (and theanine, an amino acid commonly found in tea) has been suggested as a way to augment the effectiveness of cancer treatment.

Unfortunately, most Americans eat very little omega-3 oils. They do get great quantities of omega-6s, however. For centuries, people maintained a ratio of about one-to-one—that is, one unit of omega-6 to one unit of omega-3. In the modern industrialized world, the ratio is twenty-to-one: twenty omega-6s to one omega-3. Eating such a large amount of omega 6's is almost a guarantee of disease. Very few humans can tolerate that much disease-causing fat.

Elevated Blood Sugar and Insulin

In addition to containing excess fat, processed foods also provide an abundance of simple and refined carbohydrates that are rapidly absorbed by the small intestine. These simple sugars flood the bloodstream with glucose, or blood sugar.

The body responds to this sudden rise in blood sugar by releasing great quantities of insulin, the hormone produced by the pancreas to make blood sugar available to cells. High insulin levels act as a signal to the body to store fat—both the fat in your tissues and the fat in your meal. Normally, you burn a fuel mix of about 50 percent fat and 50 percent sugar, but when blood glucose and insulin levels jump, your body attempts to burn only the sugar and store any fat in the blood and tissues. This, of course, causes weight gain and greater tissue oxidation. High insulin levels predispose a person to salt-retention and therefore high blood pressure, as well.

Many people who are overweight or obese have extremely high insulin levels. Additionally, they usually tend to be insulin-resistant, meaning their cells require greater amounts of insulin in order to absorb blood sugar. Insulin resistance is easily diagnosed by measuring the hemoglobin A1C in the blood or by the elevated "C-peptide" test, which indicates when there is an excess of insulin.

When blood sugar and insulin levels are high, the body is forced to burn only blood sugar, while it stores fat. Unfortunately, people who are insulin resistant are usually not active enough to burn all the blood sugar that's available in their bloodstreams. Any unburned sugar is stored in their bodies as fat, as well. As long as their insulin levels are high, overweight people will store fat and convert any unburned sugar to additional fat, which is why they gain weight so easily.

As if all of this was not enough, the unhealthy fat in processed foods makes cells resistant to insulin, which means the body is forced to produce more insulin to make sugar available to the cells. This combination of factors—high blood sugar, fat storage, and high insulin—is now being called insulin resistance or metabolic syndrome. Scientists now believe that insulin resistance syndrome is responsible, at least in part, for many serious illnesses, including adult-onset diabetes. There is also scientific evidence that points to insulin resistance syndrome as a contributor to breast, colon, and prostate cancers.

In the February 1999, issue of the *European Journal of Clinical Nutrition*, oncologist Betsy Stoll of St. Thomas' Hospital in London stated that one of the central causes of breast cancer throughout the West is insulin resistance syndrome. She reported that "The growth of breast cancer is favored by specific dietary fatty acids, visceral fat accumulation, and inadequate physical exercise, all of which are thought to interact in favoring the development of the insulin resistance syndrome."

A more recent study, completed in 2005 by Leslie Bernstein, PhD, found that a high level of exercise, which reduced the percent body fat, was shown to prevent breast cancer.

Of course, various fatty acids—specifically omega-6s—depress the natural immune and healing response, fueling malignancy.

You can lower blood glucose and insulin levels very rapidly by avoiding processed foods and by eating unprocessed whole grains, fresh vegetables, beans, and fruit. Such a change in your diet should also lead to weight loss. Moderate exercise also brings down both glucose and insulin levels. The single most effective answer to insulin resistance syndrome is a whole and unprocessed diet with adequate physical activity. That's also the fastest and most healthful way to lose weight, improve immunity, and feel better.

The Maximum Healing Program (see the Four-Week Program described in Part II for details), will boost your immune response, fight cancer, and lower your weight rapidly and healthfully. One of the ways it does this is by lowering insulin levels. As long as your insulin level is low, you will burn both glucose and fat, which means you will be losing weight, even while you are resting. Low insulin is one of the keys to weight loss, low oxidation levels, and a strong immune response.

All of which explains why cleaning up your system—especially through dietary change—is so important. By adopting the diet that I outline in Part II, you will dramatically lower your fat intake—both saturated fats and omega-6s. Your intake of processed foods will drop, which means your insulin levels will fall, and you'll lose weight. Lower insulin will also reduce your risk of cancer.

Fiber: Cleansing and Ridding the Body of Harmful Substances

Fiber should be viewed as binding with cholesterol, fat, and harmful hormones that promote diseases like breast cancer. Fiber independently lowers blood cholesterol. Fiber also scrubs the intestinal tract clean of stagnant and decaying waste products that have been held in pockets within the digestive tract, especially the large intestine. Those waste products can promote digestive disorders, including diverticulosis and colon cancer.

Studies have shown that fiber can reduce the incidence of diverticulosis; it can also restore the health and vitality of the colon even after diverticulosis has occurred. Other research has demonstrated that high-fiber diets reduce potentially cancerous polyps in the colon. Finally, fiber promotes healthy bowel elimination, the primary way of removing unwanted hormones and other harmful substances from the system.

As you may know, fiber can only be obtained by eating plant foods. Animal foods do not contain fiber.

Exercise: Another Cleanser

You can also cleanse your system with exercise, which improves circulation and the elimination of waste products through the breath, lymph system, and sweat glands. As I'll demonstrate in Chapter Nine, exercise improves cardiovascular fitness and respiratory and digestive function.

Exercise is one of the best detoxifying activities you can engage in. And you don't need to torture yourself in order to get fit. In fact, I do not want you to push yourself beyond your limits. Exercise must be age-appropriate. As you'll see in Chapter Nine, intense exertion provides only modest benefits. Moreover, excess exercise can depress the immune system. You were designed to be physically active, but the emphasis must be on enjoying yourself.

Making a Powerful Immune System

You don't want to just clean your system; you want to make your immune function even stronger in order to promote health and Maximum Healing. Immune boosters help you do this.

In the chapters that follow, I examine each of the major immune boosters and its effects on immune response and health. For now, allow me to summarize just some of the benefits that immune boosters can provide for your health.

Antioxidants, of which there are many, slow and sometimes stop the oxidative process. In doing so, they effectively address the underlying causes of aging and of virtually every serious illness.

Immune boosters maintain the health of cell membranes of immune cells and improve communication within immune cells. This makes immune cells better able to identify potential threats to your health. The real power of the immune system does not engage until the system recognizes the presence of an enemy.

Immune boosters improve the ability of immune cells to produce cytokines, which improve communication throughout the immune system, and make a much more coordinated and effective attack on a pathogen or cancer cell. For example, vitamin E and selenium, two antioxidants, increase production of interleukin-2 (IL-2). CD4 cells produce IL-2 in order to call out and stimulate natural killer (NK) cell activity.

Immune boosters stimulate immune cells to reproduce in greater numbers and make them more aggressive in the face of any threat to health. Immune boosters make immune cells tougher, stronger, and far more effective killers. For example, certain antioxidants—especially vitamin C and selenium—have been shown to make NK cells more aggressive, especially against cancer. Natural killer cells are among the immune system's greatest cancer fighters. They are the attack dogs of the immune system, designed to seek out and destroy nests of cancer cells, also called micrometastases. Macrophages, which attack and destroy bacteria, viruses, and cancer cells, are also made more numerous and aggressive by certain immune boosters, especially vitamin C, and by several medicinal plants, including echinacea, ginkgo biloba, shiitake mushroom, agaricus blazei, and cordyceps. Immune boosters make CD4 cells more numerous and powerful against an antigen, as well. These lymphocytes are especially stimulated by vitamin E (of the right kind).

Immune boosters reduce stress, thus controlling a powerful source of immune depression. At the same time, stress reduction techniques—such as meditation, prayer, and positive visualization—promote positive thinking, which may elevate the number of CD4 cells and make the immune response stronger.

Immune Boosting Can Make All the Difference

In the modern scientific world, we refer to certain diets, nutrients, and behaviors as "immune boosting," but in the past, medicinal foods and healing activities were basic medical tools, typical parts of the medical armamentarium. Many health-promoting activities were woven into the culture and therefore were considered second nature, and even common sense. When scientists look at traditional cultures and compare them to our own, they have found dramatic differences in disease patterns, especially in heart disease, diabetes, and cancer rates.

One of the more interesting patterns discovered among traditional cultures is that great numbers of people actually have small nests, or clusters, of cancer, but they never know it. These cancers appear, remain stable, and do not spread. Many of the people who have these cancers die late in life without ever experiencing any symptoms or signs of cancer. Only upon autopsy do doctors discover the presence of cancer.

What was keeping these cancers in check for all the years these people actually had the disease? The short answer, according to the research, is an immune-boosting diet and lifestyle. Studies have shown that the immune system actively fights these non-life-threatening cancers and keeps them in check. This is particularly true in Asia, specifically in Japan and China.

For example, it's common for Japanese men to have latent prostate cancer that never spreads, nor affects their health. These cancers never become clinically significant, meaning they never affect the lives of these men. By contrast, American men have 120-fold more clinically significant prostate cancer. In other words, the cancers in American men progress beyond the dormant stage and become life threatening. Other research has shown that when Japanese men move to Hawaii or the U.S. mainland, adopting the American diet and lifestyle, their clinical cancer rates rise to American levels.

All of this begs the question: what is present in the traditional Japanese lifestyle that protects them from this dread disease? The traditional diet of Japanese men consists of far less meat, saturated fat, and processed foods than the typical diet of American men. Japanese men also eat more whole grains, fresh vegetables, beans, and soybean products. Soybean products— including tempeh, tamari, miso, and shoyu soy sauce (shoyu is high quality soy sauce similar to tamari)—for example, contain a phytochemical called genistein that studies have shown blocks tumors from developing blood vessels. Without blood, cancer cells cannot get adequate oxygen and nutrition to survive. (See Chapter Four for more information on phytochemicals, including genistein. See Chapter Six for more information on other cancer fighters.)

A diet that is low in fat and contains a high proportion of plant foods is a powerful immune booster and cancer fighter. More and more research shows that prostate and breast cancers, under certain conditions, can remain under control, or "in situ," and thus never emerge as life-threatening. This means that the immune system recognizes the cancer, battles it consistently, and is able to keep it in check, often without the person ever knowing that a cancer is present.

In China, Dr. T. Colin Campbell and his colleagues from Cornell University found that Chinese living in rural areas had far less cancer than those living in cities. The big difference, they found, is that in the cities, people eat diets richer in saturated fat, omega-6 fatty acids, and processed foods. Consequently they are more overweight than their rural countrymen. Their health reflects this difference.

What I would like you to understand is that immune boosting is a way of life. It must become second nature to us, as it is among all traditional peoples.

As you will see in the chapters that follow, there are many immune boosters, including numerous vitamins, minerals, plant substances, medicinal foods, herbs, and immune-enhancing behaviors. It is my hope that as you incorporate these behaviors and dietary factors into your life, they will become second nature to you.

I'll conclude this chapter with another illustrative case example. One of my patients, Leon, was a thirty-six-year-old man who stood just over six feet tall and weighed a little more than four hundred pounds. Leon had a wife and two children. He worked for a local neighborhood grocery store. Before Leon became my patient, I used to go into the store from time to time and see him working. One day he turned up in my office and said he wanted to lose weight. He had heard that I advise people on diet and lifestyle. Maybe I could help him, he said.

I was only too happy to oblige. I took my standard lengthy history, asking him what he ate the day prior to his office visit for breakfast, lunch, dinner, and snacks. I also conducted a standard physical exam, an array of blood and other lab tests, and an electrocardiogram—a test that can reveal the health of the heart.

Not surprisingly, I found that he was diabetic and had heart disease. I gave him prescribed medication to help control his diabetes and heart condition, but I told him that if he followed the diet I recommended and walked every day, he might eventually be able to come off both medications.

I then described the diet and daily exercise program I wanted him to follow, the program that I have laid out in detail in Part II of this book.

For the next two years, I saw Leon regularly to check on his progress and evaluate his medication. During that time, he lost 200 pounds and, as I had promised, I took him off both medications. One day, I said to him, "Leon, what gave you the strength to lose all that weight?"

"I don't know," he said. "One day, I just decided that I didn't want to be fat anymore."

That answer was good enough for me.

CHAPTER FOUR

Antioxidants and Immunity

When most people hear the word antioxidants, they think of vitamins C, E, and beta-carotene, and they think of them in the form of vitamin pills. The truth is that there are hundreds of antioxidants. Some are commonly known vitamins and minerals; others are less well-known chemicals, found in plant foods, called carotenoids, bioflavonoids, and phytochemicals. There are literally hundreds of carotenoids and thousands of phytochemicals. A great many of them serve as antioxidants.

In fact, scientists have now identified six hundred carotenoids and up to twenty-five thousand phytochemicals (chemicals found in plants). Most of these chemicals have unknown effects on the body, but the more scientists learn about these substances, the more impressed they are with their effects on human health. With so many important substances in food, the question naturally arises: how can you possibly get all of them in optimal amounts? The answer obviously is to eat their sources, a plant-based diet—a Liv-it!—of grains, vegetables, and beans (GVB).

There are between a hundred and fifty thousand and two hundred thousand plant foods that include an enormous variety of whole grains, leaves, roots, tubers, beans, stems, fruit, seeds, and nuts. Multiple researchers have found that primitive people, who have low rates of cancer, heart disease, and other disorders, commonly eat eight hundred varieties of plant foods as part of their overall diet.

By contrast, many Americans eat only three vegetables per day, and these often include French fries, tomato in the form of ketchup, and iceberg lettuce on a hamburger. Many of these Americans think they can balance junk food diets by taking vitamin and mineral supplements. However, knowing that there are twenty-five thousand phytochemicals alone, you can easily see that no pill will ever match the nutrients found in food. Some supplements, when taken in the wrong doses, can even be harmful.

New research has shown that megadoses of vitamins may actually backfire. Even antioxidants, when taken in high doses, can trigger oxidation, turning these disease-fighting substances into disease-causing agents.

A study published in the *New England Journal of Medicine* showed just how destructive antioxidants can be when taken in the wrong doses. Researchers found that cigarette smokers who took beta-carotene supplements actually had higher rates of lung cancer than those who did not take supplements.

In fact, research has consistently shown that the greatest benefits from antioxidants come when they are taken as part of a balanced diet. Antioxidants, carotenoids, and phytochemicals work synergistically, scientists now believe. That means that they have their greatest health effect when consumed together as food. Clearly, the whole is greater than the sum of its parts. When taken individually, they can have positive or negative effects, depending on the dose, or no effect at all (See Chapter Seven for information on how to take supplements safely and effectively.) Clearly, the best way to derive maximum benefits from antioxidants and other plant substances is to eat them as part of your diet.

Plants are the primary source of antioxidants and the only source of carotenoids and phytochemicals. We should not be surprised, therefore, that researchers have found that vegetarians have significantly higher antioxidant levels—particularly of vitamin E—in their bloodstreams than meat eaters do. Animal foods are essentially devoid of antioxidants (as well as lower in potassium and magnesium and higher in sodium). When you think of antioxidants, therefore, think first of beans and grains, then of vegetables, fruits, nuts, seeds, and even tea or chocolate that is at least 85 percent cocoa.

The general rule: for adequate amounts of antioxidants and phytochemicals, eat a minimum of five servings of vegetables, fruits, legumes, and whole grains per day. Some health authorities recommend between seven and nine servings of these plant foods per day. I simply say, let your diet be organic, unprocessed whole foods and you'll be fine without the counting.

Another way to look at it: eat 95 percent unprocessed (organic whenever possible) whole grains, vegetables, beans, fruit, nuts, and seeds—a Liv-it, not a die-t. I believe that everyone should eat at least five servings of vegetables per day, at least one serving of fruit (berries for the overweight), and at least two servings of whole grains per day (fewer, or none, for the overweight).

In Chapter Eleven, I provide dietary recommendations that will give you optimal amounts of antioxidants and phytochemicals, even if you regularly eat in restaurants. As I will show, it's not difficult at all to get abundant quantities of antioxidants and phytochemicals every day. And as you will see, the health benefits of eating these foods are enormous.

Antioxidants

In addition to the three antioxidants people are most familiar with—vitamins C, E, and beta-carotene—there are vitamin B6, coenzyme Q10, glutathione, manganese, selenium, zinc, and manganese, and the amino acids L-cysteine, N-acetyl cysteine, and superoxide dismutase (SOD). Several occur naturally in the body—coenzyme Q10, L-cysteine, N-acetyl cysteine, and SOD, specifically—and are consumed largely as supplements. All the other antioxidants occur in food—primarily plant foods. So, you might be asking, what can antioxidants do for your health?

Boost Immunity

Antioxidants are powerful immune boosters. First and foremost, they prevent oxidation and the creation of radicals. In chemistry, radicals, commonly called free radicals, are atomic or molecular species with unpaired electrons. The immune systems must deal with both oxidation and free radicals. When these toxic molecules are diminished, the immune system can turn its attention to the other problems facing the body.

While all antioxidants act as free radical scavengers, vitamin C is among the strongest. A study done by Dr. Bruce Ames and his colleagues at the University of California at Berkeley showed that oxidation of the blood fat LDL (also known as oxidized LDL) ceased entirely as long as vitamin C was adequately present in the bloodstream. The researchers said that it is possible that vitamin C may be capable of "completely protecting lipids against detectable" oxidation.

In addition, antioxidants have a direct impact on the immune system itself. When consumed in adequate dosages, antioxidants boost the number and aggressiveness of virtually every type of immune cell, including CD4 lymphocytes, macrophages, granulocytes, and natural killer cells. When they have sufficient antioxidants in reserve—that is, in the bloodstream and tissues—these cells are far more effective against disease.

Vitamin C appears to be particularly adept at preventing inflammation associated with a more aggressive immune response. One of the benefits associated with decreased inflammation is a reduction in the discomforts normally associated with colds and flu. People with asthma and arthritis may also benefit, since these illnesses are associated with inflammation, especially when symptoms flare. My routine directions for the treatment of respiratory infections include taking five hundred milligrams of vitamin C three times per day for five days.

Beta-carotene appears to boost the immune system's fight against yeast infections, specifically *Candida albicans*. Astaxanthin is a strong carotenoid anti-inflammatory that has eleven times the effect of beta-carotene and 550 times that of Vitamin E. A serving of wild Alaskan sock-eye salmon has the correct dose.

A study published in the September 1994 issue of *American Journal of Clinical Nutrition* showed that a group of people over the age of sixty who took an antioxidant multivitamin every day had particularly strong immune responses to antigens. The researchers gave twenty-nine people an antioxidant combination for twelve months. They compared this test group to a control who received a sugar pill as a placebo. At six months and then twelve months into the study, they gave all the participants a skin test in which they were exposed to proteins from bacteria and fungi that cause, among other things, tuberculosis. The researchers then measured the participants' immune responses and found that the people who were given the antioxidant combination had far stronger immune responses than those who did not get the antioxidants. Those getting the antioxidants were able to fight off infection far easier, without suffering any signs of infection or disease.

"Improved immunity will lead to fewer infections," said study leader John Bogden, PhD, professor of preventive medicine and community health at the New Jersey Medical School in Newark. "It may also influence the risk of getting cancer, since the immune system plans an important role in the defense against the development of cancers."

Bogden was quick to point out that the basis for a healthy immune system is an antioxidant-rich diet. The reason: no one knows which antioxidant or combination of antioxidants will have the greatest effect on an individual. "One nutrient, like B6 or vitamin E, may help some older people, while for others it may not be either of these, but may be vitamin C. The first line of defense is a good diet based on high intake of grains, vegetables, beans, fruits, nuts, seeds, and low intake of saturated fat." (See Chapter Six for more information about cancer.)

Reduce the Risk of Heart Disease

Antioxidants prevent the oxidation of LDL particles in the blood, thus reducing atherosclerosis. People who eat antioxidant rich plant foods every day have much lower rates of heart disease, heart attacks, strokes, and high blood pressure than those who eat few vegetables, beans, grains, and fruit.

Harvard University's Nurse's Study, for instance, which has been following the health of more than eighty thousand women for over a decade, has shown that women with higher blood levels of vitamin E have lower rates of heart disease. The researchers found that women who ate five or more servings of carrots per week had 68 percent fewer strokes than those who ate carrots only once a month. Women who ate antioxidant-rich foods also suffer significantly fewer heart attacks, researchers have found.

Studies have consistently shown that vitamin C protects cholesterol from being oxidized and turned into atherosclerosis as stated in the *Cold Spring Harbor Laboratory Press,* 1992.

One study showed that as little as 180 milligrams of vitamin C per day—the amount found in two stalks of broccoli—reduced the risk of heart disease and lowered blood pressure (*Procedures of the National Academy of Sciences,* September 1993, Vol. 90, 7915–7922). Vitamin C also may increase HDL cholesterol, the good cholesterol that prevents heart attacks and strokes.

Vitamin E appears to be particularly effective at preventing atherosclerosis, the underlying cause of heart disease, and keeping arteries clear. In the Harvard Nurses study, women who took one hundred international units of vitamin E per day experienced 40 percent fewer heart attacks than those who avoided vitamin E-rich foods or vitamin E supplements.

Reduce the Risk of Cancer

Cornell University researchers have shown that Chinese who live on traditional grain-vegetable-bean (GVB) diets have the highest blood levels of antioxidants and the lowest cancer rates. While antioxidants boost all immune cells against disease, they appear to have a particularly strong effect on natural killer cells and their ability to destroy cancer cells.

A study published in the medical journal *Cancer* (March 15, 1991, Vol. 67, No. 6) reported that beta-carotene significantly improved the ability of natural killer cells to wipe out cancer cells. Other studies have shown that men who eat green, leafy, and yellow vegetables every day have higher levels of beta-carotene in their bloodstreams and lower rates of prostate cancer. Beta-carotene appears to stimulate macrophages to gobble up cancer cells and produce more tumor necrosis factor, the cancer-killing cytokine.

Research has consistently shown that people whose diets are rich in vitamin C have lower rates of breast, colon, and prostate cancers. Vitamin C reduces inflammation associated with immune responses. Chronic inflammation is now regarded as a leading cause of cancer, as well as heart and other diseases.

Reduce the Negative Effects of Aging

People who eat diets rich in antioxidants experience a much lower incidence of age-related disorders, including cataracts, arthritis, immune depression, and muscle loss. Vitamin E prevents the breakdown and wasting of muscle tissue associated with aging; supports and sustains improved fertility; protects the body from oxidative damage that causes cancer, heart disease, and cataracts; and may prevent and reduce the symptoms of arthritis, asthma, and immune deficiencies. The combination of vitamins C and

E appears to be especially effective at improving immune response and overall health in the elderly.

Antioxidants in Your Diet

Vitamin C

The recommended daily allowance (RDA) for vitamin C is sixty milligrams, but that is now widely regarded as well below what is needed. Good sources of vitamin C include broccoli (a single stalk of broccoli has more than twice the RDA for vitamin C), cantaloupe, citrus fruits, kiwi, red peppers, and strawberries.

Vitamin E

The RDA for vitamin E is ten milligrams, which scientists now believe is well below optimal levels. New research suggests that anywhere from twenty to thirty milligrams is optimal and supplements that deliver between two hundred and four hundred milligrams have been shown to be safe and effective at immune boosting. For vitamin E, two-thirds of a milligram is one international unit (IU). When buying a vitamin E supplement, be sure to get one that has all four tocopherols and all four tocotrienols.

Excellent food sources of vitamin E include whole grains, cold- or expeller-pressed vegetable oils, wheat germ, sunflower seeds, nuts, almond butter, kale, and spinach.

Beta-Carotene

There is no established RDA for beta-carotene, but optimal levels appear to be around thirty milligrams per day. I believe mixed carotenoids (with lutein, lycopene, zeaxanthin, astaxanthin, etc.) are best.

Good sources of beta-carotene or mixed carotenoids include all green, yellow, and orange vegetables and fruits, including collard greens, kale, mustard greens, dark lettuce (such as romaine), broccoli, pumpkin, squash, carrots and other root vegetables, Brussels sprouts, and virtually all colorful fruit, such as apples, pears, strawberries, blueberries, blackberries, cherries, and many others.

Antioxidant-Rich Foods

Scientists at the USDA Human Nutrition Research Center on Aging at Tufts University in Boston studied the effects of antioxidant-rich foods for each food's ability to snuff out free radicals. They then ranked the foods in five tiers according to their antioxidant powers. They also ranked the foods within each tier. For example, the foods in tier one provide the most abundant source of antioxidants available, but Concord grape juice and blueberries are far more abundant sources than, say, prunes or an orange, which are also in tier one. Prunes (which are good for preventing osteoporosis) and oranges (both tier one) are richer in antioxidants than any of the foods in tier two, however, just as the foods in tier two are more abundant in antioxidants than those in tiers three, four, and five. The foods in all five tiers are good sources of antioxidants.

Tier One: The Greatest Antioxidant Sources (listed in descending order from most to least antioxidant-rich)

- Red beans
- Whole grains
- Concord grape juice and pomegranate juice
- Blueberries
- Blackberries
- Strawberries
- Prunes
- Cranberries and a combination of cranberry and blueberry juices
- Green leafy vegetables, including collard greens, kale, and spinach
- Oranges

Tier Two: Powerful Antioxidant Sources

- Brussels sprouts
- Grapefruit juice
- Pecans
- Plums

- Apples
- Pink grapefruit
- Orange juice
- Avocado
- Red grapes
- Cranberries
- Cherries
- Cooked corn
- V-8 Cocktail juice (but high in sodium)
- Red bell peppers

Tier Three: Excellent Sources of Antioxidants

- White mushrooms
- Apple juice
- Raisins
- Onions

Tier Four: Good Sources of Antioxidants

- Eggplant
- Broccoli florets
- Cranberry juice cocktail
- Carrots
- Peach
- Banana
- Pear
- String beans
- Cauliflower
- Cantaloupe
- Apricots
- Cabbage
- Tomato
- Yellow squash

Tier Five: Adequate Sources

- Honeydew melon
- Lettuce
- Watermelon
- Cucumber
- Celery

Carotenoids: The Medicinal Power of Color in Vegetables

Carotenoids are the substances that give vegetables and fruits their rich colors. Many of the six hundred known carotenoids act as antioxidants, but researchers have now established that these chemicals are less powerful alone than when they work in harmony with each other, and with phytochemicals. Laboratory studies have shown that carotenoids have a particularly powerful effect as immune boosters and cancer fighters. Though the early research centered on beta-carotene, new and exciting studies have focused on other carotenoids, two in particular: lycopene and lutein.

Lycopene, the carotenoid that gives the red color to tomatoes, is one of the most powerful antioxidants in the food supply. New research has shown that lycopene may be protective against an array of diseases, including many forms of cancer. It appears to be particularly protective against cancers of the mouth, esophagus, stomach, colon, rectum, and prostate. One study found that women with the highest levels of lycopene in their bloodstreams were five times less likely to suffer precancerous cells and tumors of the cervix than women with the lowest levels.

Lutein, which is found in broccoli, Brussels sprouts, spinach, kale, and egg yolk, may offer significant protection against macular degeneration, a degenerative eye disorder. Macular degeneration afflicts one third of all adults over the age of seventy-five. The carotenoid astaxanthin may be even more helpful than lutein.

The following foods provide the most abundant quantities of carotenoids (in descending order):

Sources of Carotenoids

Vegetable or Fruit Source	Total Carotenoids in Micrograms
Tomato juice, canned	23,564
Kale	22,610
Collard greens	18,445
Spinach	15,385
Swiss chard	12,488
Watermelon	12,166
Carrots	11,696
Pumpkin	10,710

(Source: The *New York Times,* February 21, 1995)

Phytochemicals: Mysterious Chemicals That Heal

Perhaps the most exciting area of nutrition research concerns phytochemicals, an enormous group of plant chemicals that includes bioflavonoid, indoles, and many other substances. Many act as antioxidants, while others suppress tumor growth, prevent blood clots, and reduce inflammation.

Indoles, a group of phytochemicals, change estrogen into its more benign forms and help prevent breast cancer. The cruciferous vegetables, such as bok choy, broccoli, Brussels sprouts, cauliflower, cabbage, collard greens, kale, mustard greens, rutabaga, and turnips, are all rich in indoles.

Saponins, found in whole grains and soy products, neutralize intestinal enzymes that cause colon cancer, while chemicals called sterols, found mostly in vegetables, lower blood cholesterol levels.

Other phytochemicals, known as isoflavones or phytoestrogens, act as mild estrogens that block tumor formation, starve tumors of blood and oxygen, and act as antioxidants. Isoflavones also prevent bone loss, lower blood cholesterol levels, and block enzymes that stimulate breast cancer. Foods rich in phytoestrogens include soy products, whole grains, berries, fruits, vegetables, and flaxseeds.

One such phytoestrogen, called genistein, has been shown to stop blood vessels from attaching to tumors, according to a study reported as far back as April 1993, in the *Proceedings of the National Academy of Sciences*. In this way, genistein prevents cancer cells and tumors from getting the blood, oxygen, and nutrition they need to survive.

Virtually all whole grains, beans (isoflavones are especially concentrated in beans), and green, yellow, and orange vegetables contain isoflavones. Asian women eat large quantities of plant foods, especially soybean products that are rich in genistein. Scientists now believe that this is one of the reasons Asian women have such low breast cancer rates. In my opinion, a low percentage of body fat and regular exercise habits are also important factors.

Miso, a soybean paste that has been fermented in salt for up to two years and is often used as a Japanese soup base, is particularly rich in genistein and is loaded with gut-friendly flora. Miso can also be made from aduki beans or chickpeas, making it suitable for people who are sensitive to soy.

Since scientists discovered the importance of genistein in suppressing tumors, miso and other soybean products have become increasingly popular. Scientists now believe that miso can play an important role in the prevention of solid tumors, including those of the breast. Dr. Judah Folkmann, a longtime cancer researcher from the Harvard Medical School whose work resulted in the chemotherapy agent Avastin to prevent tumor blood vessel development, said that genistein might be an ideal form of cancer therapy. Genistein attacks the cancer cells but leaves normal cells unaffected.

Miso is rich in friendly bacteria, such as lactobacilli, which aid digestion and make nutrients more available to the small intestine. It is also a good source of protein.

Miso is bought as a paste in tubs and added simmered, but not boiled, to soups, stews, and sauces. About one-half teaspoon can be added to a bowl of soup to give it a rich, hearty flavor. I recommend use of refrigerated varieties, rather than freeze dried or pasteurized. (See Chapter Fifteen for more information on incorporating more isoflavones, including miso, into your diet.)

As powerful as all of these chemicals are, they are only part of the wondrous health-promoting substances in plant foods. Grains, vegetables, beans, fruits, nuts, and seeds are also among the richest sources of other vitamins and minerals. They are your body's sources of fiber, and the relatively small amounts of fat that they provide actually support and encourage your health.

Let's turn now to the mineral content of plant foods to see how these tiny metals that are so abundant in plants can boost your immune system and help you ward off cancer and other diseases.

CHAPTER FIVE

Minerals: Essential for Your Health

When he first came to see me, Bruce, a forty-eight-year-old computer technician, had an array of problems, including adult-onset diabetes, excess weight, high blood pressure, chronic headaches, and constipation. Among the first set of blood tests that I ordered for Bruce were a red blood cell magnesium test (RBC-magnesium), as well as blood urea nitrogen (BUN), and creatinine.

The first test, which revealed the amount of magnesium in his cells as opposed to his bloodstream, told me that he had low magnesium levels. Magnesium is essential for healthy heart, blood pressure, and bowel function. The other two evaluations, both kidney function tests, informed me that his kidney function was still within the normal range. This led me to conclude that Bruce could supplement his diet with magnesium without worrying that it would depress his heart function, which is a concern for those with reduced kidney function. (For more information on supplements and organs, such as the kidneys and heart, see Chapter Seven).

Bruce's low magnesium levels didn't surprise me at all. If there is a single group of people who have notoriously low magnesium levels, it is pre-diabetics and diabetics, especially those with adult-onset diabetes. One reason for those low levels is that adult-onset diabetics tend to eat diets that are rich in animal foods, especially fat, and low in plant foods. Their bodies use up their magnesium stores and crave additional magnesium, but their diets don't provide it. The result is low magnesium, which can cause a variety of symptoms, including anxiety, headaches, constipation, and irregular heart beat. However, many patients with low magnesium don't display recognizable symptoms. It isn't until the magnesium is replenished that the patient tells me about ten different things that have vastly improved.

Magnesium is essential for healthy heart, blood pressure, and bowel function. Another symptom of low magnesium is headaches. Bruce had all the signs. Obviously, Bruce's problems had multiple sources, most of which had to do with his diet, which was not providing enough magnesium and included too many calories (virtually all type 2 diabetics have an elevated percentage of body fat).

One of the first prescriptive steps I took with Bruce was to repeat my food mantra: "Fresh, whole and unprocessed, organic, fiber." I then gave him one of my many handout sheets describing those recommendations in detail. "Make your diet *fresh,*" I said, which means placing an emphasis on fruits and vegetables. "Be sure that it's *whole* food." Whole food means food the way it grows in the field, before man does anything to it. Examples of whole grains are brown rice, barley, millet, and quinoa. Beans are also a whole food. "Whenever possible, choose *organically grown* food." And finally, "The vast majority of your foods should contain *fiber.*" That means, of course, that most of Bruce's diet should be of plant origin, since only plants provide fiber.

I outlined my dietary recommendations in detail, going over the recommended grains, vegetables, beans, and fruits. I also included certain animal foods in limited amounts. I recommended that Bruce begin taking chelated magnesium, a three hundred-milligram capsule once per day at first and later adding a second three hundred-milligram capsule per day. I urged him to walk daily and to follow the diet as closely as possible. Two of the consequences of his new diet and daily exercise routine would be weight loss and a reduction in his blood pressure.

Bruce was already taking blood pressure medication. I added another medication, but I assured him that the exercise, weight loss, and magnesium would directly address all of his issues—his diabetes, high blood pressure, headaches, excess weight, and constipation.

In three months, Bruce was a new man. He lost weight, normalized his blood pressure, and needed less medication for his type 2 diabetes. His headaches and chronic constipation were gone. I lowered the magnesium and reduced the number of days he took the supplement.

Minerals are essential for virtually every metabolic and immune-related function. The body uses them to conduct cellular functions and build bones, muscle, nerves, organs, teeth, and connective tissues, such as ligaments and tendons. Minerals are also used to spark and conduct electrical currents along the nervous system, including the brain. All minerals come from the earth. Plants absorb minerals, which are then eaten by animals and people. Animal foods often contain significant amounts of individual minerals—iron in meat or calcium in dairy foods, for example—because animals eat plants.

Minerals are essentially tiny bits of metal. There are more than sixty different types of minerals and they are all imperishable. If you had a box full of minerals and then burned the box, all of the minerals would still be present after the fire died out. The body recycles many minerals, but twenty-two are considered essential, and they can only be derived from your diet.

The only way to ensure that you will get adequate minerals is to eat a healthy diet rich in plant foods including whole grains, fresh vegetables, and beans, with only a small amount of animal foods. Sea vegetables, such as nori, arame, wakame, and hijiki, are among the richest sources of minerals.

As long as you are eating a plant-based diet supplemented with a palm sized (your palm for you, my palm for me) serving of healthy animal foods—wild fish, bison, and free-range poultry, for instance—not more than two to four times a week, you will almost certainly maintain optimal mineral levels. I often recommend a supplement that includes minerals, especially for people who are transitioning from an unhealthy diet to a healthy regimen.

Five minerals are especially essential for your health and your immune system: calcium, iron, magnesium, selenium, and zinc.

Calcium for Healthy Bones, Teeth, and Muscle Tissue

You need calcium for strong bones, healthy teeth, and muscle tissue. As an electrolyte, calcium helps conduct electrical charges throughout the nervous system and the heart. It is essential for healthy heart function and balanced blood pressure.

How much calcium do you need? That is one of the most controversial subjects among nutritionists today. Many nutritionists believe that a calcium deficiency in modern America and certain parts of Europe is causing an unprecedented epidemic of osteoporosis and other disorders.

The Food and Nutrition Board of the National Academy of Sciences recommends that Americans eat at least eight hundred milligrams of calcium per day. The Board urges women at risk of osteoporosis to consume between twelve hundred milligrams to fifteen hundred milligrams per day, which in my opinion is a lot of calcium.

Personally, I strongly doubt that any culture in the last five hundred years has consumed that much calcium per day.

Around the world, people do not get anywhere near the amounts of calcium recommended by American health authorities, yet they experience very low rates of osteoporosis. Researchers have found that most populations consume between three hundred and five hundred milligrams of calcium daily. The World Health Organization recommends between four hundred and five hundred milligrams per day, which is about what people on traditional diets get. The average Chinese person, for example, consumes 544 milligrams of calcium per day, yet the Chinese have exceedingly low rates of osteoporosis.

It's worth noting that osteoporosis is a distinctly modern problem. It is also a distinctly Western problem. People in Asia, Eastern Europe, the Middle East, Africa, and in developing countries do not experience the high rates of osteoporosis that Americans do, even though American health authorities stress the consumption of enormous amounts of calcium. Something is obviously wrong with this picture.

That "something" is protein, especially protein from animal sources. Once it is consumed, animal protein increases the acid levels of your bloodstream. Your body wants to keep your blood at a balanced pH, leaning slightly toward alkalinity.

That means that when acid levels increase, your body wants to immediately alkalize, or buffer them. It does this by releasing its own natural alkalizing or buffering agent, namely the phosphorous from within your bones. Unfortunately, when the phosphorous is released from the body, so too is the calcium. That loose calcium is excreted in the urine and over time can lead to osteoporosis and kidney stones. That, of course, makes your bones weaker.

Researchers have found that the more protein you eat, the more phosphorous and calcium your bones lose. That's the finding from numerous studies, including one published in the *New England Journal of Medicine* (1994). Another study done by Harvard University's Mark Hegsted, PhD, and published in the *Journal of Nutrition* (1981), found that doubling protein intake increased urinary calcium losses by as much as 50 percent.

Writing in the professional journal, *Dietitian's Edge* (May/June 2001), Belinda S. O'Connell, MS, RD, reported, "We know that dietary protein intake influences urinary calcium losses with each gram of protein increasing urinary calcium losses by one [to] one and a half milligrams. This means that a person who is consuming a high-protein diet requires more calcium in his or her diet to maintain calcium balance than someone who eats less protein. In situations where dietary calcium intake is suboptimal, a high-protein diet may further worsen calcium imbalances and increase the risk of osteoporosis."

Think about what the Atkins and South Beach diets are doing.

Traditional populations do not eat the amounts of animal protein that we do in the United States. In fact, low intake of animal protein may be one of the more important elements protecting the Chinese from osteoporosis.

The average Chinese eats just over sixty-four grams (a little more than two ounces) of protein per day, sixty of which are from plant sources. Compare that to the average American who eats between ninety and 120 grams of protein daily, only twenty-seven grams of which come from plant sources. We eat more protein, and the great majority of it comes from animal food sources. That's why Americans have osteoporosis and the Chinese don't.

Health authorities routinely suggest that you prevent osteoporosis by drinking milk—it's supposed to "do the body good"—and eating milk products, such as cheese and yogurt. Unfortunately, the little bit of research on this subject has not been supportive of that recommendation.

As far back as 1985, the *American Journal of Clinical Nutrition* published a study that investigated how much calcium was gained or lost in women who drank milk. The study compared two groups of women, one that drank three additional eight-ounce glasses of skim milk per day, with one that drank no additional milk. Both groups consumed the same amount of calcium per day, which was fifteen hundred milligrams.

The researchers studied how much calcium the women in the two groups would retain. After one year, the researchers found that the milk drinkers had slightly greater calcium losses than the non-milk drinkers. The authors concluded that, "The protein content of the supplement (the skim milk) may have a negative effect on calcium balance, possibly through an increase in kidney losses of calcium or through a direct effect on bone reabsorption."

This finding was consistent with other research. Writing in the journal *Science* (April 22, 1994), the dean of the school of nutrition at Harvard University, Walter Willet, MD, PhD, reported the following. "Adult populations with low fracture rates generally consume few dairy products and have low calcium intakes. Milk and other dairy products may not be directly equivalent to calcium from supplements, as these foods contain a substantial amount of protein, which can enhance renal [kidney] calcium losses."

How Much Protein Do You Really Need?

Protein is used by the body for cell replacement and repair, meaning it is one of the essential building blocks of cells, organs, and tissues. All whole, unprocessed plant foods provide protein, often in optimal amounts. As long as you eat a diet composed largely of unprocessed plant foods, you will not have a protein deficiency. The real concern, as I've said before, is excess protein, which is far easier to fall victim to than deficiencies in protein.

After lengthy observation, the World Health Organization initially recommended that at least 2.5 percent of calories come from protein. Believe it or not, there are traditional populations that survive on that little protein. Having established that percentage as a minimum, the World Health Organization scientists then doubled that number, stating that all men, women, and children around the world should get at least 5 percent of their calories from protein. Next, they went a step further. The scientists recommended that pregnant women should get 6 percent and nursing women should get 7 percent of their calories from protein.

In fact, as long as you are eating unprocessed plant foods with grains and beans, it's pretty hard not to meet—and exceed—the WHO standards, as the chart below shows.

Percent of Calories Derived from Protein

Rice	8
Corn	12
Pinto beans	24
Broccoli	43
Cauliflower	33
Zucchini	17
Orange	9
Strawberries	8

I recommend that your primary sources of protein come from non-animal plant foods. If you exercise frequently, my recommendations allow up to one animal food entrée—preferably one low in fat—every other day. I suggest that you limit the size of that portion to three to four ounces, about the size of a deck of cards or the size of your *palm,* not your whole hand. That will give you a diet that's around 15 percent total calories from protein, which is more than enough protein to meet your needs. A six-ounce portion of meat, fish, or egg entrée is acceptable if these foods are consumed only twice a week.

In short, you needn't worry about getting too little protein. Most people today—especially women—should be more concerned about getting too much.

Exercise for Healthy Bones

One of the best things you can do for your skeleton is exercise. Especially important are weight-bearing exercises.

Bone is very active tissue; it's always naturally breaking down and restoring itself. As long as the raw materials are present—and virtually everyone has them—that restoration usually leaves bone in a stronger, firmer, and more resilient state. The restoration process occurs more rapidly when you exercise regularly. People as old as one hundred have been found to produce stronger bones after regular weight-bearing exercise.

Exercise physiologists recommend that you exercise at least four days a week. For those concerned with osteoporosis, that exercise routine should include a thirty-minute walk and twice weekly weight training sessions of fifteen minutes each. (See Chapter Eight for more information about exercise.)

Other Factors to Keep Your Skeleton Strong

Several other factors are important in preventing osteoporosis:

- Get adequate vitamin D. Half of all Americans are deficient in this fat-soluble (stored in your tissues) vitamin. Twenty minutes of sunlight per day, even on an overcast day, in the warmer six months of the year will give you all the vitamin D you need. Be sure to wear sunscreen with adequate protection (minimum SPF 30) when you go outdoors between eleven o'clock in the morning and two o'clock in the afternoon.
- Drink alcohol only in moderation. I recommend that people limit themselves to four drinks per week or less. Alcohol weakens bone. Alcoholics suffer far more fractures—including deadly hip fractures—than do people who are not alcoholics, and that isn't just from being too wobbly.
- Talk to your doctor about limiting the use of steroid hormone drugs as much as possible. Steroids can cause bone loss. Prednisone and the inhaled corticosteroid asthma drugs can promote the onset of osteoporosis and possibly cataracts. Discuss these drugs and osteoporosis-preventing treatments with your doctor if you require these medications.
- Limit caffeine consumption. Coffee and cola beverages contain caffeine and phosphate salts, both of which may promote calcium loss.
- Limit sodium intake. Use modest amounts of salt in cooking. Try not to use salt as a condiment at the table.
- Consider a bone density DEXA (and not a QCT) scan. This is a

non-invasive test that can provide highly accurate information about the condition of your bones. Such information can help you design a new exercise regimen to strengthen specific bones that may be thinning; and can inform you if you need more vitamin D or medications. (More helpful information on vitamin D can be found at www.mercola.com.)

- If you are a woman with small bones, you should be especially careful about osteoporosis. It's important for you to follow all the advice provided here. Limit your intake of protein and get regular exercise, adequate sunlight, and adequate calcium (eight hundred milligrams per day for most).

Milk and the Immune System

It's worth considering the impact of milk products on your health for reasons other than building healthy bones. For many people, cow's milk consumption can have an especially adverse effect on the immune system.

The immune system can recognize milk proteins—called bovine albumin peptide—as antigens, or disease-causing agents. In a study published in the *New England Journal of Medicine* (July 1992), researchers at Johns Hopkins University showed that the proteins in cow's milk could attach themselves to tissues throughout the body, including those of the pancreas, the organ that produces insulin. Insulin makes blood sugar available to cells. Without it, cells are deprived of fuel and eventually die.

In sensitive children, proteins found in cow's milk may trigger an immune response. Immune cells produce antibodies that attack both the bovine proteins, as well as the pancreas. In the process, the insulin-producing beta cells of the pancreas are destroyed, thus rendering the pancreas unable to produce insulin. This condition, known as juvenile (type 1 or insulin-dependent) diabetes, requires insulin injections for the rest of one's life in order to survive.

This same process may be one of the causes of rheumatoid arthritis, scientists now believe. Milk proteins may attach themselves to the synovial tissues between the joints, which in turn are attacked by the immune system, causing the standard array of symptoms, including inflammation, pain, redness, fever, and deformity.

The proteins in cow's milk are also a leading source of allergies in sensitive children. Studies have shown that cow's milk can cause asthma, bedwetting, chronic runny nose, ear infections, and eczema.

Of course, there is also the problem of lactose intolerance, which is the inability to digest the sugar in milk products, known as lactose. Much of the world is lactose intolerant. In fact, in most traditional cultures from Asia to North and South America to certain parts of Europe, people naturally lose lactase, the enzyme needed to digest lactose, after the age of three or four. This means, of course, that they lose the ability to digest milk after they have been weaned.

The old aphorism that it's both unnatural and unhealthy for one animal to drink another animal's milk seems to apply to humans. Human breast milk derives only 5 percent of its calories from protein, while whole cow's milk and skim milk derive 21 percent and 41 percent of calories from protein, respectively. That's a lot of protein, especially when you consider that many children experience adverse reactions to proteins in cow's milk. It's also disheartening to think of all the women drinking milk every day to protect their skeletons, when in fact, they may very well be promoting calcium loss and accelerating the onset of osteoporosis by consuming an excess of protein.

It's inconceivable for many people in the West to think about life without cow's milk, but it's worth noting that approximately 70 percent of the world's population does not drink cow's milk or eat milk products. Interestingly, osteoporosis is most common among milk-drinking nations. Or, as Dr. Willet mentioned in the *Science* article quoted previously, those populations with low fracture rates generally consume little or no milk products.

Where Can You Get Calcium?

The first thing people ask me when I suggest that milk products may be giving them more trouble than benefit is, "Where can I get my calcium?"

Actually, calcium is abundant in green vegetables, as well as many other sources. A cup of milk contains about three hundred milligrams of poorly absorbed calcium. Here are some alternatives to milk as a source of calcium:

- Almonds (one-third cup): 130 milligrams
- Beans (one cup, cooked): 100 milligrams
- Bok choy (one cup, cooked): 250 milligrams
- Broccoli (one cup, fresh): 140 milligrams
- Collard greens (one cup, cooked): 360 milligrams
- Kale (one cup, cooked): 210 milligrams
- Herring (three and a half ounces): 250 milligrams
- Mackerel (three and a half ounces): 300 milligrams
- Mineral water (calcium quantity varies by brand)
- Salmon (three and a half ounces): 290 milligrams
- Sardines (sixteen ounces): 480 milligrams
- Sesame seeds (half cup): 80 milligrams
- Sea vegetables or seaweed (See Chapter Ten for more on sea vegetables and Part II for information on how to easily incorporate these foods into your diet.)
- Supplements (See Chapter Seven on supplements.)
- Tofu (four ounces, about the size of a deck of cards): 150 milligrams

Iron: Not as Simple as We Used to Think

You probably remember a time when health authorities emphasized the importance of getting adequate iron. Well, iron is still an important mineral, but we now know that iron can also be dangerous when consumed in excess.

Iron is a pro-oxidative mineral—it triggers the creation of free radicals—when consumed in the high doses common in supplements. Excess iron consumption has been linked to liver cancer and other diseases.

You only need ten milligrams of iron per day, which is pretty easy to obtain through a healthy diet. In fact, supplement guides often don't include a recommendation for iron consumption because of iron's tendency to promote oxidation. In any event, no iron supplement should exceed ten to fifteen milligrams.

Deficiencies and excesses of iron do impact the immune system, however. Deficiencies weaken the overall immune system's ability to fight infections.

Excesses tend to be far more dangerous. Excess iron can cause the following:

- Weakened natural killer cell activity.
- Increased numbers and aggressiveness of CD8, or suppresser T-cells. CD8 cells, you will recall, turn off the immune system. CD8 cells tend to be in excess in the immune systems of people infected with HIV or with full blown AIDS.
- High levels of oxidants, free radical formation, and an increased risk of liver cancer, as well as other forms of cancer.

If you are a menstruating woman with low iron, I believe you are in all probability allergic to dairy products. Some experts tell us allergic reaction to dairy can cause excessive menstrual bleeding and, as a result, iron loss. Hence, removing *all* dairy products from your diet will likely reduce menstrual losses and clear up the anemia.

For all of these reasons, I recommend that you get your iron from a healthy diet, unless your doctor has determined that you are deficient in iron and need a supplement. Your doctor can monitor your iron levels while you are taking the supplement and take you off the iron pills once your iron levels have stabilized.

Good sources of iron include shrimp and fish; green and leafy vegetables; tofu; whole grains, especially millet; beans; and nuts. I'd rather you get your iron by cooking in a cast-iron pot than by eating meat or poultry.

Magnesium

Magnesium works with more than more than a hundred enzymes in your body to create an incredible array of essential biological reactions. It is essential for healthy heart function, balanced blood pressure, protein formation, and the creation of healthy DNA. Magnesium reduces insulin resistance in diabetics and is essential for the body to utilize calcium. People with low magnesium can experience arrhythmia, asthma, kidney stones, and high blood pressure. Muscles that do not have adequate magnesium easily go into spasm and cramp.

As for the immune system, magnesium is needed to create what are called adhesion molecules or integrins. Immune cells adhere to these molecules and use as transportation throughout the system—they're essentially a subway system. Adhesion molecules also help immune cells stick, or adhere, in great numbers to the places in the body where infection may lie or disease is concentrated.

Optimal levels of magnesium are 350 milligrams per day for men and 280 milligrams per day for women. Good sources of magnesium include whole grains, especially barley, brown rice, and millet; leafy green vegetables such as collard greens, kale, broccoli; beans; nuts; and fruit (GVB does it once again).

Selenium

Selenium, an important antioxidant, is now being recognized for a host of important health benefits. It is an immune booster and a major reducer of oxidation and free radical formation. While these effects are important, it is selenium's ability to prevent cancer—and possibly treat the disease—that researchers are most excited about today. First, let's look at its effects on the immune system.

Selenium has been shown to boost the number and aggressiveness of CD4 T-helper and natural killer cells. It also increases production of interferon and boosts antibody production from B-cells. When you add the fact that selenium is proving to be an especially important cancer fighter, you begin to understand why scientists are so excited about this mineral. Information published in 2007 showed that selenium-supplemented HIV patients faired better than those without the selenium.

A ten-year study conducted by Cornell researchers Gerald Combs Jr., PhD, and Larry Clark, MD, of more than thirteen hundred people found that those who took two hundred micrograms of selenium daily had 37 percent fewer instances of new cancer and less than half the cancer deaths than those who were given a placebo, or non-therapeutic pill. Combs and Clark found that the study group—those receiving the selenium—had half the rate of prostate cancer and greater than a third fewer incidences of lung and colon cancer.

Other research has shown that selenium inhibits cancer growth in people with existing tumors. It has also proven to be protective against breast cancer and in 2006 was shown to slow HIV progression.

Since the Cornell researchers reported their findings, the National Cancer Institute (NCI) has begun large-scale studies on selenium's effects on the rates of prostate cancer and on colon cancer.

Selenium is available in a wide array of foods, including nuts (especially Brazil and walnuts), wheat and whole-wheat products (bread and noodles, for example), brown rice, barley, oats, fish, shellfish, and sunflower seeds. One or two Brazil nuts eaten five times per week provide a sufficient supply of selenium.

Zinc

Zinc is one of the most powerful immune boosters in the food supply. It is essential for the healthy development of the thymus gland, which incubates and grows T-cells. When zinc levels are low, the thymus atrophies and produces fewer and far less aggressive T-cells, or lymphocytes. Fortunately, when zinc is replenished, the thymus tissue returns to normal and the number and aggressiveness of immune cells is restored.

Low zinc has a weakening effect on immune cells that is independent of the thymus gland, however. Zinc deficiencies make CD4 cells fewer in number and less aggressive in the face of an antigen, and B-cells do not produce optimal levels of antibodies

People with low zinc levels have significantly higher rates of infections. This is especially true of infants and children. According to the April 1994 issue of the *Journal of Intellectual Disability Research,* one study followed two groups of infants, one receiving a zinc supplement and the other receiving a placebo. The supplemented group had fewer infections, higher blood levels of lymphocytes, and better weight gain than the group receiving the placebo.

Other disorders associated with zinc deficiency include: weight loss, loss of the sense of taste and smell, amenorrhea (failure to menstruate), testicular retardation, rashes, dwarfism, and increased susceptibility to infection.

Increased zinc consumption helps the body overcome the symptoms of a common cold quicker than if zinc levels are not increased.

Animal studies have shown that zinc boosts the body's immune response against Candida infection.

Like selenium, zinc slows the growth of cancer cells and tumors.

Interestingly, excesses of zinc clearly depress immune function. Studies have shown that excess zinc intake weakens CD4 cells and granulocytes, promotes nausea, vomiting, bleeding, and abdominal pain. A study of men with HIV found that those who took excesses of zinc were more likely to progress to full-blown AIDS.

As with other minerals, it is critical to balance your intake of zinc—to get enough, but not too much. Optimal amounts of zinc range from ten to fifteen milligrams per day, but scientists discourage anyone from taking amounts greater than thirty milligrams per day. In 2007 it was reported that high zinc intake was associated with an enlarged prostate.

Zinc, sometimes called the "intelligence mineral," is available in a wide range of foods, including beans; whole grains such as millet; shellfish (especially shrimp, crab, and oysters); red meat; turkey; and chicken.

Minerals are essential for your good health, and those I've discussed in this chapter are among the most important of them. You need them all, and the best way to get them is to eat a plant-based diet, supplemented with low-fat wild or free-range animal foods.

The dietary approach I describe in Part II of this book will ensure that you get all the minerals you need. (See Chapter Seven for information on how you can supplement your diet safely and optimally.)

CHAPTER SIX

Healing Foods That Boost Immunity and Fight Cancer

L onnie, now nearly sixty years of age, is a woman with whom I have worked for many years. One of Lonnie's most obvious characteristics is her vivaciousness. She's full of life, energy, and optimism. If you don't know anything about Lonnie's past medical history, you would never guess that this woman was once at death's door.

In the early 1990s, Lonnie was diagnosed with breast cancer. She had long been suffering from fibrocystic breasts. A tumor was discovered, which initially was determined to be benign. She was forty-four years old at the time. The February following her initial diagnosis, she started to suffer severe pain that ran from her left breast down through her left arm. She knew something was very wrong.

Lonnie's doctors performed a biopsy and discovered the tumor was malignant. She underwent a radical mastectomy that surgically removed her entire left breast and seven lymph nodes. Six months of chemotherapy followed, as well as six weeks of radiation treatment. She received Tamoxifen, a drug to reduce and control her estrogen levels. Estrogen, the female hormone, is a risk factor for causing breast cancer, especially when it is elevated, as it was with Lonnie.

During the course of her treatment, Lonnie's coworker, Linda, gave her an article that appeared in *Life* magazine about a medical doctor who had overcome cancer. The article was based on the book *Recalled by Life: The Story of My Recovery from Cancer* by Anthony J. Sattilaro, MD, with Tom Monte. Dr. Sattilaro was president of Methodist Hospital in Philadelphia, Pennsylvania. He had been diagnosed with prostate cancer that had spread throughout his body. After being told that he had only eighteen months to live, he adopted a macrobiotic diet and began a spiritual transformation that eventually led to his full recovery. The diet Sattilaro followed was composed mostly of whole grains, fresh vegetables, beans, sea vegetables, various soups, condiments, fruit, and small amounts of fish (quite similar to what I recommend in this book).

Lonnie thought nothing of the article at the time. She was undergoing treatment and believed that her cancer was under control. However, she began suffering from severe menstrual cramping, stabbing pains, and bloating. These symptoms continued for the next three years, and eventually, a bone scan revealed cancer in several sites in her pelvis and spine. She also developed numerous tumors in her ovaries and uterus.

Doctors performed a hysterectomy. They also wanted Lonnie to undergo chemotherapy and radiation, but she decided to undergo just the radiation. The chemotherapy, she believed, was too toxic for her to bear and, in any case, she learned it was not likely to send her disease into remission. Lonnie went through another round of radiation treatments, but they did not stop her disease. She continued to have cancerous tumors in her pelvis and spine.

Shortly after Lonnie began her radiation treatments, she woke up one morning with the memory of the *Life* magazine article about Dr. Sattilaro. She could not remember the doctor's name, or the hospital where he worked, but her friend Linda not only remembered the article, but also gave Lonnie a copy of it.

After reading the article again, she began to explore books about macrobiotics, including *The Macrobiotic Way,* by Michio Kushi, the leading American teacher of macrobiotics. Lonnie read the book and decided to begin the diet. She traveled to Boston, where Kushi taught, and met with a macrobiotic counselor. The counselor outlined a diet and offered encouragement, telling Lonnie that he believed following such a diet would help her overcome her disease. Lonnie returned home and adopted the macrobiotic diet with fervor.

She did not stop with a change in diet, however. She was raised in a devoutly religious Italian family. Prayer and meditation were already a fundamental part of her life, but now she prayed as she had never prayed before. Her way of praying was noteworthy, I believe, because she didn't just ask that God miraculously heal her. She prayed that God would lead her to the solution to her illness. She promised to surrender to the Divine Guidance, as she perceived it. She decided she would adopt any method or approach that she intuitively felt was being sent to her from God. In other words, Lonnie was willing to change and do anything she felt guided to do in order to become well.

Having established a healthy way of eating and a daily ritual of prayer and meditation, Lonnie began to seek out the best alternative healing advice she could find. That led her to Bernie Siegel, MD, well-known author of *Love, Medicine, and Miracles,* the groundbreaking book that revealed how people were using mental, emotional, and spiritual approaches to overcome severe illnesses, including cancer.

Lonnie began attending Dr. Siegel's seminars. During one such program, this statement struck a chord with her: "We have the power to make ourselves sick. We also have the power to make ourselves well. In order to do that, we have to realize that each of us has both a death wish and a life wish. Which one is stronger in us now, we must ask ourselves? How do those respective wishes influence our daily behavior? How do they influence our choices in life, especially the choices of how we treat ourselves and take care of our bodies, minds, and spirits?"

"That made sense to me," Lonnie recalled. "What Dr. Siegel was saying was that we have to make our wish for health practical. It has to influence what we do every day. You can't just think you want health and then go out and do all these things that are no good for you. If you eat badly, then something other than your wish for health is going to determine the outcome of your illness."

After he spoke that day, Dr. Siegel asked everyone to sit together in a circle. As fate would have it, he sat next to Lonnie.

"Dr. Siegel talked for a little while, and then he put his hand on my back," Lonnie recalled. "He touched my spine, right on the place where I had a tumor. I was so moved. I felt energy pass between us and right into my spine. I was so touched, and I felt so lucky to be sitting next to him."

Meanwhile, Lonnie's health was very much in crisis. She had lost a great deal of weight and had become extremely weak. She had little or no appetite and could hardly hold down food. And her grain-vegetable-bean diet only made it worse, it seemed, because she didn't like the food at all. "I didn't know how to prepare the food, and it tasted terrible to me," Lonnie recalled.

Lonnie's coworker was her ever-present cheerleader. Linda had also adopted the macrobiotic diet to support Lonnie, and the two would often eat together.

"Oh, Lonnie, isn't this food delicious?" Linda would say to Lonnie, hoping to encourage her to eat more. But Lonnie's appreciation for the food was anything but enthusiastic.

"I would be gagging on the miso soup and sea vegetables," Lonnie recalled. "I told Linda, dying is one thing, but starving to death is a hell of a way to go."

Lonnie was only half-joking, but every night she would pray that God would tell her whether or not she should stick to this diet, along with all the other things she was doing for herself.

About three months after she had adopted the macrobiotic diet, Lonnie was awakened in the middle of the night with a terrible pain in her spine. The tumor in her back had become red, hot, and swollen. Apparently, the swelling was pressing on a nerve, and it was causing tremendous pain.

"I didn't know what to do," Lonnie said. "I called Linda and told her what was going on. She reminded me that the macrobiotic philosophy maintained that once you adopt the diet, you start to eliminate, or discharge, the toxins that support the disease. 'Maybe your body is discharging,' Linda suggested.

"'Oh, Linda,' I said. 'What if the tumor is getting bigger and the disease is progressing? I don't know if I can stand this kind of pain.'"

A few days later, however, all the redness, swelling, and pain had disappeared. In fact, there seemed to be no sign of any tumor on her spine.

"That was a turning point," Lonnie said. "After that, I started to feel better and better. My energy levels returned, my skin became brighter and healthier, and I started to gain weight. I felt like I had come through something, and I was on the other side."

In September 1997, Lonnie had a bone scan that revealed that her tumors were 25 percent smaller than they had been just nine months earlier. Her doctors could not explain why her condition appeared to be improving. Her doctor told her, "Lonnie, you look great. You're obviously making progress. How do you feel?"

"Well, Doc," Lonnie said, "If this is dying, I highly recommend it."

A bone scan a year later revealed that her tumors had nearly disappeared. A subsequent scan revealed no sign of cancer anywhere in her body.

Today, Lonnie teaches natural foods and macrobiotic cooking in the greater Hartford area. Lonnie and I work together; she provides meals and cooking classes to many of my patients. She is an inspiration to them because she reveals what is possible, even when someone appears to be at death's door.

How You Can Protect Yourself from Cancer

No other illness is feared as much as cancer, and with good reason. Each year, cancer kills about nearly half a million people in the United States, making it a close second to heart disease, the leading cause of death among Americans. The most common cancers, of course, are those of the lung, colon, breast, prostate, pancreas, and ovary, which collectively comprise about 60 percent of all cancers.

Most cancers are caused by a combination of environmental pollutants, unhealthy diet and lifestyle, and genetic predisposition. Yet, despite the terrible fears people have of this disease, it has been my experience that only a minority of the population is willing to make the changes in behavior to protect themselves from illness. I believe that if all of us focused on our fear more clearly and honestly, more people would change—and do it gladly. Even more people would change if they realized how easy it is to get out of real danger.

Another thing people don't realize is that the same unhealthy diet and lifestyle that create the most common forms of cancer also give rise to heart disease, adult-onset diabetes, high blood pressure, and other degenerative diseases. In fact, the original title of this book was to be *All Diseases Are One*.

The leading killer diseases all have the same causes—the standard American diet (SAD) and lifestyle. If your genetic makeup predisposes you to cancer, as opposed to heart disease, that's likely to be the illness that you will get if you eat a diet that's rich in fat and processed foods and don't exercise. If you're predisposed to heart disease, you're more likely to have a heart attack than to be diagnosed with breast or prostate cancer. The meat, dairy, and sugar diet attacks your weaknesses and brings on the illnesses to which you are the most vulnerable. It is a formula for sickness, as research has consistently shown.

Scientists have found that between 60 and 90 percent of cancers have external causes. I believe the most important of these causes is diet, which influences your percentage of body fat.

I know what you're thinking: "I thought smoking was the most significant environmental cause of cancer."

Actually, it's the combination of cigarette smoking and unhealthy diet that represents the most powerful poison people can take into their bodies. The combination of smoking and a high-fat diet is particularly lethal. A study reported in a 1987 issue of the *Journal of the National Cancer Institute* (79:631) showed that cigarette smokers on low-fat diets had lower rates of lung cancer than smokers on high-fat diets. Other studies have supported this finding.

The Japanese are among the highest per capita cigarette smokers in world, but they also have one of the lowest lung cancer rates in the world. Why is this so? Scientists now believe that the traditional Japanese diet, which is low in fat and high in plant foods, protects the Japanese, to a point, from lung cancer.

Twenty out of every hundred thousand Japanese people die of lung cancer each year. In the United States, where Americans eat an average of fourteen hundred calories of fat per day, the death rate is fifty-five people per hundred thousand. That's more than double the Japanese experience.

I distinguish between the "traditional" Japanese diet—the one that emerged from the Japanese culture thousands of years ago—and the one that's taking hold of the Japanese people today. The modern Japanese are adopting a more Western-style diet that is richer in fat and animal foods and lower in plants, which very likely is the primary reason their cancer rates are going up. Those Japanese who eat the way their ancestors did are still eating mostly unprocessed whole foods and very little animal fat.

During the last four decades, research has consistently shown that diet either contributes to—or directly causes—most of the common cancers we see today. The single biggest poison in the diet, of course, is fat (and I say, only half humorously, anything else that isn't included in the Food Mantra's grains, vegetables, beans, fruit, and some wild game). Among the many studies showing that fat increases the rates of the common cancers is reported in a 1992 issue of the medical journal *The Lancet* (340:162). That study found that fat contributes directly to cancers of the breast, prostate, and colon.

Scientists have been reporting the relationship between the American diet and common cancers for decades. Among the best-known scientific and government bodies that initiated dietary recommendations and still urge Americans to change their diets in order to prevent cancer are: the Senate Select Committee on Nutrition and Human Needs (1977), the National Cancer Institute (1979), the National Academy of Sciences (1982), the American Cancer Society (1984), and the Surgeon General of the United States (1988).

All of these health authorities have recommended for many years that we reduce our intake of fat, animal foods, and processed foods, and increase our intake of unprocessed whole plant foods.

Getting the Fat Out

In Chapter Three, I said that you should do two things to boost your immune system and overall health: clean up your inner environment and eat foods that boost your immune and cancer-fighting systems.

In this chapter, I offer specific dietary and herbal advice as it relates to cancer, immune function, and overall health and the promotion of Maximum Healing. But before I get to those substances that directly fight cancer and boost immune function, I have to address one of the major causes of cancer: dietary fat. Let's begin with the job of cleaning up your system and significantly reducing your intake of fat.

Fat intake is linked to every major cancer, including lung, breast, prostate, ovarian, colon, and pancreatic. Fat triggers the onset of cancer, and fuels its growth once it manifests. It does both of these things in several ways.

First, fat is a huge free radical producer. It breaks down and deforms the DNA of cells, causing some cells to start reproducing without regard to the overall health of the body. After cancer manifests, these free radicals support the life of cancerous cells and tumors. In other words, cancer depends on free radicals. That's why high-fat diets are so toxic and lethal to people who already have cancer.

Fat weakens your immune system: as fat supports the life of the cancer, it weakens your immune system at the same time. This gives the incipient cancer cell the environmental conditions it needs to proliferate.

Excess dietary fat dramatically elevates production of the reproductive hormones, namely estrogen and testosterone. High estrogen levels have long been shown to promote cancers of the breast, uterus, and ovaries. High levels of a metabolized form of testosterone, called dihydrotesterone, have been shown to cause both swelling of the prostate and prostate cancer.

One of the ways fat promotes the onset of breast cancer, for example, is by adding weight to the body. Fat cells produce hormones that are converted by the body into estrogen, which has been shown to promote cancer. Fat also stimulates malignancy by secreting cytokines (cell movers).

A study published in the *Journal of the National Cancer Institute* (1996, Vol. 88:650–660), reported that overweight and obese women have twice the risk of contracting breast cancer than women who are at their ideal weight or lower. Moreover, women who lost weight reduced their risk considerably.

"Weight loss was consistently associated with reduced risk," said one of the lead researchers on the study, Dr. Regina Ziegler of the National Institutes of Health.

Women in their forties and fifties who lost excess weight just ten years earlier—that is, in their thirties and forties—cut their risk of contracting breast cancer in half. On the other hand, women who gained eleven or more pounds in their fifties had three times the risk of contracting breast cancer than women who did not gain those pounds.

Researchers speculate that increased body fat leads to breast cancer by increasing estrogen levels, particularly estradiol, which has been shown to promote the onset of breast cancer and then feed tumors after they manifest. Studies have shown that when estrogen levels fall, tumors shrink.

Plant-based, high-fiber, low-fat diets have been shown to lower estradiol levels by 40 percent.

Fat also increases blood cholesterol levels, which have been shown to feed cancer cells once they manifest. Studies have shown that when cholesterol levels have been lowered significantly (below 120 milligrams per deciliter), cancer cells begin to die. This finding, however, could be the old statistical problem of "coexistence versus correlation." Was it the diet that achieved both results? Or was the low cholesterol part of the anti-cancer regimen itself?

That is the basis for Tamoxifen. A study by Dr. James Carter and his colleagues at the Tulane School of Public Health in New Orleans reported that men with prostate cancer who followed a macrobiotic diet lived longer than men who received standard medical treatment. Among the things Dr. Carter found was that everyone who extended their lives on a macrobiotic diet experienced dramatic reductions in blood cholesterol levels. Once again, is this "true, true and related or unrelated?" Macrobiotics is a form of what I recommend: an organic unprocessed whole foods GVB Liv-it.

The macrobiotic diet is low in fat and rich in antioxidants, phytochemicals, carotenoids, and fiber—all-important in the body's fight against cancer.

In fact, dramatic reductions in fat and blood cholesterol seem to be among the keys to protecting yourself against cancer, or in fighting the disease once it manifests.

Numerous studies have shown that, once cancer develops, people on a low-fat, plant-based diet have much longer life spans than those who eat a high-fat diet. This finding was dramatically illustrated in a recent study conducted by Dr. James Hebert and his colleagues at the University of Massachusetts Medical School in Worcester.

Hebert followed 472 women, all of whom had been diagnosed with breast cancer by doctors at Memorial Sloan-Kettering Cancer Center in New York. All the women underwent extensive questioning regarding their dietary and lifestyle habits. The scientists followed the women's health for the next ten years. The study findings were important for every woman in America.

Hebert and his coworkers found that:

- Diets richer in calories dramatically increase the likelihood of recurrence of breast cancer, especially for premenopausal women.

Women who had not yet entered menopause were 45 percent more likely to suffer a recurrence for every thousand additional calories they consumed over their ideal calorie intake. As it turned out, most of those additional calories were from fat consumption.

- Butter and margarine are particularly lethal. Women who ate these foods were 67 percent more likely to suffer recurrence of the disease.
- Meat, especially liver and bacon, can be deadly. Those women who ate these foods regularly were twice as likely to suffer recurrence.
- Vegetables and fruits rich in vitamin C can save a woman's *life*. Postmenopausal women who ate vitamin C-rich vegetables and fruit every day had half the risk of recurrence than those who didn't.
- Lifetime exercise also proved important for reducing body fat, cancer risk, and recurrence risks.

Many other studies have implied or directly supported these same findings. Excess consumption of dietary fat is a trigger for cancer and a promoter of the disease after it appears. This information about "lifetime exercise" preventing cancer was just published "anew" in 2005.

Types of Fats and Their Effects on Health

There are four types of fats, two of which are particularly toxic. Those four types of fats are described below.

- Saturated fats are found primarily in animal foods, such as red meat and dairy products. (Fish tend to be richer in polyunsaturated fats, including the health-promoting omega-3 fatty acids.) Saturated fats raise blood cholesterol levels, specifically the "bad" LDL cholesterol (low density lipoprotein). These fats can affect gene transcription that causes higher blood cholesterol and can also become oxidized free radical producers. They create the atherosclerosis (hardening of the arteries) that leads to angina, heart attack, angioplasty, and stroke. They are immune depressing and cancer promoting.

- Trans fats, also known as partially hydrogenated vegetable oils, are found primarily in processed foods, such as margarines, muffins, pastries, doughnuts, and precooked and packaged foods. They raise levels of triglycerides, one of the blood fats. They rapidly oxidize, giving rise to floods of free radicals. They are immune suppressing and cancer promoting. New Federal labeling now requires that these levels be listed on commercial food products and in 2006 New York City began to eliminate them in restaurant fare.

- Polyunsaturated fats are found in vegetables, seeds, nuts, grains, and cold-water fish. Polyunsaturated fats are also found in vegetable oils, such as safflower, corn, and sunflower oils. Polyunsaturated fats lower blood cholesterol, especially when eaten in the quantities provided by food. When eaten in excess, such as in excessive quantities of vegetable oils, they have been found to promote the onset and life of cancer.

- A fraction of polyunsaturated fats, called omega-3 fatty acids, are immune boosting. Omega-3 fatty acids also have been shown to prevent cancer and promote the body's ability to fight cancer. Omega-3s are found in cold-water fish including cod, flounder, haddock, halibut, scrod, salmon, mackerel, sardines, swordfish, and tuna, as well as in olive oil and many seeds and nuts.

- Monounsaturated fats are found in olive oil and are highest in macadamia nut oil. But the wisdom for the use of olive oil may have to do with its high content of anti-inflammatory polyphenols. Olive oil contents also raise nitric oxide and those with oleuropein improve immunity and blood pressure. These fats do not affect blood cholesterol, except to create small increases in the good cholesterol called HDL (high density lipoprotein). Monounsaturated fats have not been shown to weaken immune response or promote cancer. Studies have consistently shown that olive oil may reduce your risk of heart disease including irregular heartbeats. Olive oil does not break down rapidly, as other oils do, which means it is resistant to oxidation. Olive oil is also a rich source of antioxidants and phytochemicals.

All fats provide nine calories per gram and can raise your percentage of body fat, which is associated with an increased risk of heart disease, adult-onset diabetes, high blood pressure, stroke, and certain cancers.

Fish are excellent sources of the healthy polyunsaturated fats and especially health-promoting omega-3 fatty acids, which have been shown to boost immune response and fight cancer. In general, fish are low in overall fat, and the fat they provide is mostly polyunsaturated omega-3s. With very few exceptions, fish are low in saturated fat. The chart below provides the amount of total fat and saturated fat found in selected types of fish.

Fat Found in Fish

Fish (3-½-ounce serving)	Total fat (in grams)	Saturated fat (in grams)
Bass	5	1
Bluefish	6	1(can be high in harmful PCBs)
Carp	7	1
Cod	1	1 (less than 1)
Flounder	2	1
Haddock	1	1
Halibut	3	1
Herring	12	3
Mackerel	18	4
Orange roughy	9	1
Red snapper	2	1
Salmon	11	2 (choose wild over farm-raised)
Sea Bass	3	1 (Chilean is endangered)
Shad	18	6
Shark	6	1
Swordfish	5	1 (High in mercury)
Trout (rainbow)	4	1
Tuna (bluefin)	6	2 (High in mercury)
Tuna (yellowfin)	1	1

The dietary program I offer in Part II of this book is low in fat, although it allows certain vegetable oils in healthful quantities. Among the most important keys to good health is this: avoid saturated fats, trans fatty acids, and even a lot of fat. This means avoiding—or at the very least minimizing—your intake of animal foods and processed fare. Eat polyunsaturated and monounsaturated fats in limited quantities. Think in terms of grains, vegetables, beans (GVB), fruit, nuts, and seeds.

The healthiest sources of polyunsaturated fats are nuts, unprocessed whole grains, and fish. Olive and macadamia oils are the preferred source of monounsaturated fats. My program not only lowers your overall fat intake, but changes the composition of fats, shifting you away from saturated and trans fats to healthful quantities of poly and monounsaturated fats. That's a big step toward a stronger immune system, prevention of cancer and other major illnesses, and greater overall health.

Foods That Fight Cancer

Let's begin our exploration of the foods, nutrients, and herbs that prevent cancer and promote good health by looking at the big picture. Although many people say that they are afraid of cancer, most do not make the diet and lifestyle changes that would protect them from this illness, as well as many others.

If you add just a few other immune boosters, such as exercise, healing foods and herbs, and some relaxation techniques, you will have created a lifestyle that results in health. With good health, you can achieve your life's goals. Health is the foundation for a long, productive, fulfilled, and happy life. What else can you ask for?

I say all of this because I don't want you to think that you should eat better just to stave off a dreaded disease—though that's a good reason in and of itself. There are a lot of benefits to good health, as I am sure you know. And those benefits don't end with just the avoidance of disease. Still, avoiding cancer and other serious illnesses is a goal for which it's worth making changes. Good health is the foundation of human freedom and, in light of today's high medical costs, health certainly creates (or at least helps to prevent the loss of) wealth.

A Very Important Caveat

No one should treat him or herself medically. For those who are interested in using diet, herbs, and supplements as an adjunct treatment for disease, including cancer, I strongly urge you to consult with your physician or other healthcare provider before taking anything, including the herbs listed here or the supplements described in Chapter Nine. Your healthcare provider will advise you accordingly or refer you to appropriate counselors. Always keep your doctor informed of any herbal remedies or supplements you are taking as these substances can interact with medications and throw off blood test results, which may cause your doctor to misdiagnose your condition or mistakenly alter your treatment.

There is no reason not to share your actions with your physician. If your doctor doesn't support you in your search for answers, find a physician who will. While initial research condemned Complementary Alternative Integrative Medicine (CAIM), much of it was done with the wrong doses or forms of supplements. Current research has found significant scientific evidence to support CAIM's usefulness. Anyone who dismisses it as quackery today is simply not up to date on the current research.

Here are some of the foods in my Maximum Healing Program that can help protect you against cancer and other forms of disease.

Whole Grains: The Basis of a Cancer-Prevention Diet

Whole grains, such as brown rice, millet, barley, buckwheat, oats, amaranth, quinoa, and teff are rich in immune-boosting nutrition and provide abundant amounts of fiber. Here's a short summary of just some of the nutrients in a few selected whole grains.

Amaranth, a tiny seed-like grain, is rich in calcium, iron, folic acid, and magnesium, and is highest in protein. It has a delicious, earthy flavor and contains no gluten, making it appropriate for those with wheat allergies (Celiac Disease). It is cooked by boiling for fifteen minutes. Check out our website, www.thepmc.org, for further guidance.

Barley provides soluble fiber, which lowers blood cholesterol. It also provides significant amounts of folic acid, magnesium, phosphorus, potassium, and zinc. Barley is how gladiators became so muscular; they were called "barley men," and the word "burly" comes from "barley." Weight lifters would do well to choose barley over whey, meat, protein shakes, and creatine.

Brown rice, also rich in soluble fiber, is a good source of B vitamins such as thiamine and niacin, as well as iron, phosphorus, and magnesium.

Buckwheat, also known as kasha, is an abundant source of selenium. It's also a good source of protein, riboflavin, calcium, and magnesium. Buckwheat is one of many quick-cooking grains, taking just fifteen minutes to cook.

Millet provides a rich supply of B vitamins, magnesium, copper, iron, and protein. It can be boiled and ready in twenty-five minutes. It is gluten-free and great for digestion.

Oats are remarkably rich in protein, iron, manganese, copper, folic acid, vitamin E, and zinc. They are great for skin, immune function, and digestion. Rolled oats are ready in about six minutes, steel-cut in twenty, and whole in thirty-plus minutes of boiling time. Oats are high in calories and, like all grains, will help prevent unwanted weight loss.

Many consider quinoa a super-grain for its abundant supply of protein, potassium, riboflavin, magnesium, zinc, copper, manganese, and folic acid. Like amaranth (and teff), quinoa is takes fifteen minutes to cook and contains no gluten.

The fiber in grains not only reduces cholesterol but also draws many cancer-promoting substances out of the body. Among the most important of these are estrogen and dihydrotestosterone, the form of testosterone that promotes enlargement of the prostate and prostate cancer.

Cruciferous Vegetables

Cruciferous vegetables include broccoli, cabbage, collard greens, kale, Brussels sprouts, mustard greens, and watercress. They contain an array of powerful cancer-fighting and immune-boosting substances, starting with a compound called sulforaphane, which stimulates the body's detoxifying mechanisms, causing the body to cleanse itself of cancer-promoting substances.

According to scientists at Johns Hopkins University, sulforaphane also triggers the body's production of anticancer substances that directly fight the disease. In laboratory studies at Johns Hopkins, 74 percent of animals given sulforaphane were protected from getting cancer after being injected with a drug that creates mammary (breast) tumors. Numerous others studies have consistently supported the finding that broccoli and other cruciferous vegetables contain powerful cancer-protective chemicals.

Scientists at Johns Hopkins say they are still some distance from creating a drug based on this compound, but they have very clear advice in the meantime. "We eat more broccoli at home, and I certainly tell my friends to do the same," said Dr. Gary H. Posner, one of the Johns Hopkins researchers who discovered the cancer-fighting effects of sulforaphane.

This is proving to be sage advice, in light of a recent study done at Fred Hutchinson Cancer Research Center in Seattle. The study found that men who eat at least three servings of vegetables daily are half as likely to contract prostate cancer than men who fail to get three servings of veggies per day. "And when we compared relative potency, vegetables from the cruciferous family, like broccoli and cabbage, reduced the risk even further," said Dr. Alan Kristal, one of the researchers in the study. The scientist rigorously examined the eating habits of 1,230 men in the Seattle area between the ages of forty and sixty-four. Overall vegetable consumption provided strong protection against prostrate cancer, but the cruciferous vegetables were the strongest.

The study, published in the January 2000 issue of the *Journal of the National Cancer Institute,* found that the cruciferous vegetables provided greater protection for men than for women.

"At any given level of total vegetable consumption, as the percent of cruciferous vegetables increased, the prostate cancer risk decreased," Dr. Kristal told Reuters news service.

Rather than naming any single compound in the vegetables, the researchers maintained that it was the abundance of the multiple phytochemicals within the vegetables that combined to offer such protection. These and other chemicals trigger compounds that are particularly active in the prostate. At this point, scientists do not know how these substances prevent cancer, but the results, they say, speak for themselves.

In addition to sulforaphane, other compounds discovered in the cruciferous family have been shown to protect against cancer. One such compound, known as phenyl ethyl isothiocyanate (PEITC), has been shown in animal studies to inhibit the creation of lung tumors in animals injected with a powerful tobacco-specific carcinogen.

These vegetables also contain other cancer-fighters known as indoles, which may inhibit or inactivate cancer-causing estrogens, especially those that affect breast tissue. Animal studies have shown that indoles trigger the production of substances that protect breast tissue when exposed to carcinogens and estrogens.

In addition, cruciferous vegetables contain hundreds of carotenoids and phytochemicals that promote immune function and fight cancer.

Another group of vegetables that may contain cancer fighters is the umbelliferous family, which includes parsley, celery, parsnips, and carrots. Researchers at the National Cancer Institute are studying vegetables closely because, as one scientist said, "These vegetables contain a great variety of phytochemicals."

Beans, Soybeans, and Soybean Products

Beans are luscious, delicious, and abundantly nutritious. They are not just adequate sources of protein, but are the richest sources of protein in the vegetable kingdom. They contain soluble fiber, which lowers blood cholesterol levels, and they provide B vitamins, beta-carotene and other carotenoids, phytochemicals, calcium, phosphorus, iron, potassium, and complex carbohydrates. They are the food group with the highest antioxidant content.

Today, scientists are discovering that we have only scratched the surface in terms of the nutritional value of beans. Some beans contain substances known as isoflavones, or plant-estrogens that dock onto the cell membrane's estrogen receptor sites. These receptors would otherwise be occupied by estradiol, the type of estrogen that deforms DNA and promotes cancer. Researchers now believe that high consumption of beans and bean products may explain why some groups of women have exceedingly low rates of breast cancer. Two such groups are Hispanic and Japanese women.

Researchers at the American Health Foundation studied the eating habits of Hispanic women and found that generally they eat twice the quantity of beans that Caucasian women do. In fact, beans and rice are eaten almost daily by a great percentage of Hispanic women who follow their traditional diet.

I recommend to my patients that in addition to eating beans they also include in their diets, moderate, not large, quantities of soy products such as tempeh, tamari, and miso, and a limited amount tofu, which is less desirable because it is highly processed. Like yogurt, tempeh, tamari, and miso all contain living organisms. Tamari and miso are high in salt and should, therefore, be used sparingly. For some people soy may be difficult to digest.

Beans and soy products contain protease inhibitors that keep animal proteins from promoting the creation of tumors. Studies have shown that animal proteins, when consumed at the levels common in the standard American diet, can trigger the malignant process. I believe that excess protein (and sugar) consumption, especially animal proteins, can support the life of cancer as well. Protease inhibitors also interfere with cancer-cell proliferation, even when the disease is established in the body (see Yehudith Birk's 2003 text, *Plant Protease Inhibitors*).

Among the most powerful of the anticancer beans are soybeans and soybean products, which make up a significant portion of the Japanese diet. Not only do Japanese women have far lower incidences of breast cancer than American women, but also those Japanese who do contract breast cancer live significantly longer after diagnosis than American women with breast cancer.

Now scientists believe they know one reason why such disparities exist. Soybeans and soybean products contain a substance called genistein, a phytochemical that blocks blood vessels from attaching themselves to tumors. Malignant tumors, like all other tissues, need blood, oxygen, and nutrients in order to survive. An important step in their survival is a process called angiogenesis, which occurs when blood vessels attach themselves to tumors and provide oxygen and nutrition to malignant cells. Genistein prevents this from occurring. This anti-angiogenic effect deprives cancerous tissue from getting blood and oxygen, essentially suffocating tumors long before they become large enough to threaten a person's life. The antiangiogenesis ability of genistein was first reported in the April 1993 *Proceedings of the National Academy of Sciences.*

Among the soybean products that contain genistein are soybeans, such as edamame (whole soybeans that are now widely available in supermarkets and Japanese restaurants throughout the United States); tofu or soybean curd; tempeh (a fermented soybean patty that tops my list of recommended soy foods); naturally aged and fermented shoyu or soy sauce; miso, an aged and fermented soybean paste that is used as a base for soups, stews, and sauces; and tamari (similar to soy sauce), the salty liquid that flows off the miso.

Numerous studies have shown that Japanese who eat miso soup every day—a soup composed of soybean miso, vegetables, and seaweed—experience 33 percent less cancer than those who never eat it.

Harvard University's Judah Folkmann, MD, who has studied angiogenesis for many years, has said that genistein might be an ideal form of cancer therapy. Genistein attacks the cancer cells but leaves normal cells unaffected.

Bean and soybean products are not only protective against breast cancer, but also all reproductive cancers, including ovarian, uterine, and prostate cancer. I highly recommend including miso soup, tempeh, edamame, shoyu, tamari, and just a little tofu in your diet. In Part II, I will show how these foods can be utilized in daily cooking.

Mushrooms

Mushrooms have long been thought of as nutritional lightweights. They are certainly delicious, and they add a lot to the flavor of a meal, but only recently have scientists awakened to their immense healing powers. Mushrooms, particularly four Japanese mushrooms, contain an array of potent polysaccharides (glucans)—long chains of sugars—that fight viral and bacterial infection, lower blood cholesterol, boost immune function, and fight cancer. The four mushrooms that provide particularly strong health-enhancing effects are shiitake, enoki, maitake, and reishi. I also recommend cordyceps and agaricus, but I don't recommend the common "button" mushrooms. Here's a closer look.

Shiitake (Genus Lentinula)

This wide, flat-capped mushroom originated in Asia and is now widely available in natural food stores and restaurants throughout the United States. Studies have shown that shiitake contains medicinal compounds that can be used to treat high blood cholesterol, high blood pressure, diabetes, and cancer.

One study showed that women who ate ninety grams of shiitake mushrooms (a three-and-a-half-ounce serving) daily for one week experienced a reduction in their blood cholesterol of between 9 and 12 percent.

Shiitake contain a polysaccharide called lentinan that has been shown to catalyze macrophages and natural killer cells to kill cancer cells and tumors in cancer patients. Japanese scientists recently approved the substance as a chemotherapy agent against cancer. Studies at the U.S. National Cancer Institute have confirmed shiitake's anticancer effects. Now scientists at the University of California–Davis Cancer Center in Sacramento are studying shiitake as a possible form of treatment for prostate cancer.

Shiitake has also been shown to be a powerful immune booster. Scientists at Japan's Yamaguchi University School of Medicine have found that shiitake extract protected cells against the destruction normally caused by HIV infection. The scientists went on to recommend that shiitake be used in conjunction with other AIDS treatments.

Goro Chihara, a leading lentinan researcher at Japan's Basic Research Laboratories, Ajinomoto Co., Inc., Kawasaki, says that lentinan ". . . prolongs the life span of patients with advanced and recurrent stomach, colorectal, and breast cancer."

Another compound in shiitake, called cortinelin, has been found to be an effective broad-spectrum antibiotic. Substances known as sulfides in shiitake can kill ringworm, fungus, and other bacteria that infect the skin. Conducting a Web search on www.google.com yields some interesting sites on medicinal mushrooms.

Reishi (Ganoderma Lucidum)

Recent studies have suggested that reishi mushrooms may almost live up to their folklore, which denotes them as "herb of spiritual potency" and "mushroom of immortality." Much of the research done on them to date has been laboratory studies on animals, but the results are so consistent that scientists believe similar results will occur in humans.

Research has shown that reishi causes lymphocytes to multiply rapidly in the presence of an antigen. It also promotes production of cytokines and tumor necrosis factor, which attacks cancer cells.

Reishi lowers blood cholesterol, lowers blood pressure, reduces asthma attacks, calms nerves, acts as a sleep-inducing agent (when cooked in water and drunk as a tea), and has anti-inflammatory powers. Since chronic inflammation is an important element in the cause of cancer, it may reduce one's risk of cancer, as well.

In a recent study, two thousand people in China with bronchitis and bronchial asthma were prescribed a pill containing reishi syrup. Within two weeks, 60 to 90 percent claimed their bronchitis or asthma had significantly improved.

Reishi is available dried and as a nutritional supplement, in liquid and solid forms, in most natural foods and health food stores.

Maitake (Grifola Frondosa)

Maitake is being studied extensively as an immune booster, a treatment for high blood pressure, and a cancer-fighter. Animal studies on maitake have shown that the polysaccharides they contain cause tumor reduction and increase the strength and aggression of immune cells. Other studies have suggested that eating maitake regularly may lower high blood pressure and help control diabetes.

Enoki (Flammulina Veluptipes)

A tiny mushroom, but one that packs a strong, delicious flavor, enoki may also be a powerful cancer fighter. Japanese farmers who grow the mushroom—and presumably eat it regularly—have significantly lower rates of cancer than those who live around them, researchers have found. Enoki contains substantial amounts of fiber, iron, and vitamin C. These mushrooms are available in stores that sell exotic varieties. Boil or steam them with other vegetables, or cook them in soups and stews.

Fiber: Powerful Protection, Especially Against Breast Cancer

Whole grains, fresh vegetables, beans, and fruit are all rich in fiber. Plant foods are the only sources of fiber, of course. Animal foods do not contain fiber.

Fiber is indigestible "roughage." It binds cholesterol, estrogens, and testosterone and helps to flush them out of your system. Bowel elimination is the primary way hormones are eliminated from the body. A high-fiber, low-fat diet is the key to balanced hormones.

A study published in the *New England Journal of Medicine* reported that vegetarian women who eat high-fiber diets eliminate two to three times more estrogen in their stool than non-vegetarians.

A high-fiber, low-fat diet was shown to reduce estrogen levels in a group of postmenopausal women by 50 percent. That's an astounding reduction, especially when you consider that research has shown that reducing estrogen by just 17 percent appears to reduce the risk of breast cancer four- to five fold.

Other Foods That Contain Cancer-Fighting Compounds

Numerous other plant foods have been shown to deliver cancer-fighting substances that have only recently begun to be studied.

Fruit, especially oranges, lemons, and grapefruit contain a substance called limonene that has been shown to shrink mammary tumors in laboratory animals, according to researchers at the University of Wisconsin. A minimum of one serving per day is recommended. It's worth noting, however, that people who take chemotherapy for cancer should avoid grapefruit because it shuts down the liver's phase one detoxification system and makes chemotherapy less effective. Turmeric and chili, both immune boosters, do the same thing, they also shut down the liver's phase one detoxification, so both should be avoided while on chemotherapy.

Flaxseeds (*not* flax oil) provide powerful protection against prostate, breast, and colon cancer.

Flaxseeds contain several anticancer substances, among them lignans, steroid-like substances that are a form of phytoestrogens, which have been shown to inhibit tumor growth. Lignans, like other plant forms of phytoestrogens, boost immune function and help the body fight cancer, including prostate and breast cancers.

Flaxseeds are particularly rich in alpha-linolenic acid (ALA), one of the omega-3 fatty acids that act as cancer-protectors. ALA is converted to DHA/EPA, but if you take a supplement, use DHA or distilled fish oil, both of which are ready for use by the body. Research at the National Cancer Institute has shown that alpha-linolenic acid may block the cancer-stimulating action of prostaglandins, hormone-like substances that fuel cancer growth. Flaxseeds also have been shown to protect colon tissue from carcinogens.

The most potent form of flaxseeds is the fresh, crushed, whole seed. Golden and brown flax are preferred over flax oil or yellow seeds. If you use flaxseeds, grind them fresh and use within two days of grinding.

Garlic and Onions

Both garlic and onions contain substances called thiols that promote cellular and liver detoxification. Among those compounds is a substance called allicin that researchers say acts as an anti-viral and antibacterial agent. Both garlic and onions also contain selenium, a known cancer fighter and strong antioxidant.

Garlic also offers significant protection against cancer. Laboratory evidence combined with epidemiological studies done by Chinese and Italian researchers suggest that garlic may be one of the reasons these populations have low rates of stomach, intestinal, and rectal cancers.

Researchers at the National Cancer Institute who have been studying garlic for decades maintain that it inhibits cancer cell reproduction and tumor growth. Garlic may block the tumor-promoting effects of prostaglandins, as well.

According to Michael Wargovich, MD, professor of medicine at the MD Anderson Cancer Center in Houston, Texas, garlic enhances the liver's ability to recognize carcinogens and transform them into harmless substances.

Some of garlic's compounds are more effective when eaten raw; others are better when cooked. Onions contain many of the same compounds as garlic, just in weaker quantities.

Use garlic and onions in cooking, salad, and vegetable medleys. Garlic can be roasted and spread on bread like butter. I recommend eating garlic two to four times per week.

Tea

Increasingly, evidence shows that both black and green teas are powerful immune boosters and cancer fighters.

Tea contains an abundance of antioxidants, bioflavonoids, indoles, and a powerful health-promoting substance called catechins that early research suggests may protect people against a wide array of cancers. So abundant are the antioxidants in tea that researchers are increasingly viewing it as an "antioxidant soup."

Tufts University scientists found that one cup of black or green tea has greater ability to protect the body against one of the most common free radicals, the peroxyl radical, than half a cup of broccoli. It beats the same amount of carrots, spinach, or strawberries at neutralizing the peroxyl radical, as well.

Obviously, I am not advocating eating fewer vegetables, which contain so many phytochemicals and carotenoids that tea does not, but the research shows that tea adds something special to the traditional "coffee break."

A study in China found that tea drinkers had 60 percent less cancer of the esophagus than non-tea drinkers. However, for those who drank scalding hot tea, the risk went up. A study of thirty-five thousand women in Iowa found that those who drank at least two cups of tea a day had 60 percent less kidney and bladder cancer and 32 percent less esophageal and colon cancer than those who didn't drink tea.

In the Netherlands, studies have shown that people who drink tea daily cut their risk of a fatal heart attack in half.

Tea contains substances known as polyphenols that may block the transformation of normal cells into malignant ones, according to C. S. Yang, a researcher who has studied tea at Rutgers University in Piscataway, New Jersey. Animal studies have shown that tea inhibits the formation of cancer cells.

Numerous studies are just beginning to study tea's effects on breast and other cancers. In the meantime, it's worth considering giving up that morning cup of coffee for two or three cups of tea.

All of this information on plant foods adds up to a single, overpowering fact: food can be powerful medicine, when it's used in the right way.

There is nothing in the medical arsenal that can equal the natural healing properties of plant foods.

On the other hand, if you eat the Standard American Diet (SAD) diet, high in fat, sugar, processed with little or no fiber, the effects of those poisons take their toll. And it becomes more and more difficult for medical doctors to overcome those toxic effects.

The power to protect your body, and even heal it, lies to a great extent with you and your actions. You have the opportunity to give your body the best medicine you can at least three times a day. Add some of the other immune boosters, including herbs and supplements, described in the next chapter, and you will be on your way to better health and all that good health can give you.

Here's another case history that I think you will find interesting:

William, a fifty-year-old man, was a lifelong meat eater and chronic sufferer of constipation. Some months before coming to me, he had surgery on his colon to remove a couple of large polyps, mushroom-like growths. Research has shown that the presence of colon polyps significantly raises the risk of contracting colon cancer. Most polyps are noncancerous, but many become cancerous.

William's surgeon noted in his report that he did not remove all of William's polyps, only the largest and most problematic. However, William needed regular colonoscopies—usually performed using "conscious sedation," which means you are asleep but wakeable.

The procedure involves insertion of a long, flexible, fiber-optic instrument into the colon to view the inside of the intestine. Colonoscopies are recommended for everyone age fifty or older, but they may be done earlier for people with a family history of colon cancer or those who are prone to develop polyps or colon cancer. William's father died of colon cancer.

Nearly a hundred and fifty thousand Americans get colon cancer each year, and approximately sixty thousand will die from it. It is estimated that six million Americans alive today will die of colon cancer.

Colon cancer is most common in industrialized nations where diets include lots of meat, saturated fat, and processed foods that are low in fiber. As Denis Burkitt, the famed Irish surgeon and researcher who studied the health of Africans, reported, colon diseases of all kinds are rare among people who eat a high-fiber diet. Much depends on the environment within the colon. The more animal foods a person eats, particularly red meat, the higher the level of carcinogens and bile acids in the intestinal tract. These carcinogens and acids corrode the cells within the intestinal lining, and the polyp itself, and increase the risk of cancer.

The September 6, 1989 issue of the *Journal of the National Cancer Institute* (81:1290) reported that a high-fiber diet reduced the size and number of colon polyps in people with a genetic disorder that causes them to produce polyps in their large intestine. This study was consistent with other reports showing that a high-fiber diet not only prevents the onset of colon polyps, but it also reduces the size and number of existing polyps.

In my consultation with William, I told him about this research and recommended that he follow my high-fiber, high-nutrient diet. William followed the diet to the letter.

One year later, a colonoscopy revealed no sign of polyps in his colon. Because this was the first colonoscopy that I had ordered on William, I could not say with certainty that his polyps disappeared on my diet. All I could do was rely on the surgeon's statement that no polyps were still present.

Nevertheless, many of William's other health indicators significantly improved. He now had regular, healthy bowel movements. He lost weight and reported experiencing a dramatic improvement in his energy levels. No matter what the status of his polyps was, he was clearly healthier in many ways, including in regards to his intestinal health.

CHAPTER SEVEN

A Guide to Using Herbs and Supplements to Boost Health

"Where do I start? Which substances should I take? How do I tell the difference between various brands offering the same vitamin or mineral?"

These are some of the questions that may go through your mind as you consider supplements.

Then there are the questions of dosage and frequency. "Should I take supplements and herbs every day? How much of a nutrient should I take?"

There is a seemingly endless array of supplements available, and it can be confusing trying to figure out which you should take, how much you should take, and how often you should take them. You may wonder if these substances are worth their high price or whether or not a particular substance is right for your body or condition.

If you have taken vitamin and mineral supplements in the past, you know that very often these substances color your urine, which means that some or all of the supplement may be eliminated from your body. That makes most people wonder whether any of the stuff that's in the bottle even remained in their bloodstreams and tissues. "Is it doing the job that I bought the stuff for in the first place?" you might ask.

That's a good question.

I have been investigating and prescribing herbs and supplements for more than twenty years. I have confronted all of these questions and many others in my medical practice. Here I have tried to provide a safe, easy-to-follow guide to supplements and herbs. Rather than throwing a lot of recommendations at you—and then expecting you to ferret out the right substance in your natural foods store—I have provided a general prescription for what to take when specific problems arise.

Here I'll address:

- Daily maintenance of immune support and protection against disease
- Enhanced immune boosting and cancer fighting
- Heart disease and lowering cholesterol
- Prostate disorders
- Asthma, allergies, nasal congestion, and colds
- Headaches
- Stronger bones, joints, and arthritis
- Improved digestion
- Mind, memory, and emotional support

For each problem, I have recommended a set of supplements and herbs. Whenever possible, I have also given a brand name for an herbal or nutrient supplement. I do this because I have found that the quality of herbs and supplements vary greatly and have determined that these brands I recommend provide the highest quality products. I have no economic relationship with any of these manufacturers. This is not to say that there aren't other fine products on the market. I simply don't know how their quality stacks up to that offered by the brands I have recommended.

Healthy Diet and Power Foods Are the Foundation

Again, your primary source of nutrition should be food. Only a health-promoting diet will ensure that your body will get the wide spectrum of nutrients it needs.

Once you have a sound dietary foundation, as outlined in the previous chapters, you can supplement your diet with important nutrients and herbs. These supplements can maximize the strength of your defenses and target specific conditions, such as heart disease, prostate problems, or allergies.

The substances recommended below are safe and can be used without ongoing medical supervision. However, be sure to provide your physician with a list of all the herbs and supplements you are taking. You may even want to show him or her the bottles each supplement comes in. In my own medical practice, I use many more supplements than those listed below, but most of those require monitoring of patients so that I can adjust the dosage and frequency when needed.

A Note on Dosage and Frequency

The purpose of herbs and supplements is to give your health a boost. These substances should be considered mild forms of drugs. They often serve as catalysts, which is one of the reasons we take them. We want them to create certain positive effects.

Typically, supplement manufacturers recommend that supplements be taken daily. I have found, however, that if herbs and supplements are taken daily, they start to lose their power to affect your body. Your body will develop a tolerance for them, the same way it develops a tolerance for caffeine, alcohol, and drugs. Eventually, higher doses are needed to create the same results. In order to avoid this problem, I recommend that supplements be taken only for limited amounts of time, in staggered doses. In most cases, I recommend that supplements be taken as directed on the package for fourteen to thirty days.

After the initial fourteen to thirty days are over, I recommend that the daily dosage be reduced by half and that you take the supplement only four days a week: Monday, Tuesday, Thursday, and Friday. Avoid taking the supplement on Wednesday and the weekend. I use the abbreviation "WWO" to indicate "Wednesdays and the weekend off." This gives your body a chance to restore its normal, baseline pattern so that it will be restimulated by the supplement when you resume taking it on Monday. Based on my experience with literally thousands of patients, I have found that this maintains sensitivity to the product and sustains the kinds of results you want to get from the supplement.

Vitamin and Mineral Supplements for Daily Maintenance of High Immunity

There are occasions when we start to feel a bit rundown and want to take an herbal or nutrient supplement to boost our immune defenses. During these times, you know you need something extra, but you may not know where to turn. Here, I have provided a recommendations for individual nutrients, namely vitamins C and E, to be taken individually or together (see Chapter Four for more information on antioxidants).

Vitamin C

Take five hundred milligrams of vitamin C, two or three times a day, four or five days a week. There are many good manufacturers of vitamin C, including MegaFood, Rainbow Light, Source Natural, and NOW brands.

Vitamin E

Take vitamin E four or five days a week. Take only natural vitamin E that contains all four of tocopherols and four tocotrienols, specifically the alpha, beta, gamma, and delta forms of both. Avoid synthetic E, as indicated by "acetate" or "succinate" as these forms are not well assimilated by the body, and therefore are excreted without being utilized making them a waste of money. Carlson's, NOW, MegaFood, and GNC brands all provide the full spectrum tocopherols with tocotrienols

Vitamin-Mineral Formulas

Vitamins and minerals work best when taken together, so taking a combination supplement is preferable to taking vitamins C and E and other antioxidants separately.

Current research confirms that vitamins, minerals, carotenoids, and phytochemicals work synergistically to create an even greater effect than individual nutrients can create alone. For example, a study appearing in the May 1991 issue of the *Journal of Age and Aging* found that one hundred milligrams of vitamin C boosted immune function, but the positive effects on immune defenses were far greater when vitamin C was combined with vitamin E and beta-carotene.

I recommend a one-a-day formula, as well as an antioxidant formula. Both can be taken with my standard approach: take the one-a-day in the morning and the antioxidant formula in the evening on Monday, Tuesday, Thursday, and Friday, with Wednesday and the weekends off (WWO).

For a multivitamin, I recommend MegaFood Iron Free One Per Day Multivitamin, a potent, high quality, food-extracted (derived from food)

formula that provides a wide spectrum of vitamins and minerals, taken WWO.

For an antioxidant formula, I recommend MegaFood Antioxidants, another food-based product that is very potent, easily assimilated, and of the highest quality. Among the immune-boosting nutrients it contains are vitamins C and E; minerals include zinc and selenium. This should also be taken WWO.

Emer'gen-C, produced by Alacer Corp., contains a wide array of vitamins and minerals. It comes in powder form, in many different flavors, and is easily assimilated. Take five hundred milligrams three times a day for five days for colds, flu, and sinus or lung infections.

I recommend Carotenoid Complex by Country Life for eye, mouth, tongue, esophageal, and urinary bladder issues. Take it WWO.

Herbs for Immune Boosting and/or Cancer Fighting

The herbs listed below can significantly strengthen your immune defenses. I recommend that they be used whenever you are battling any sort of infection. Some are better used for a cold or flu; others are highly effective against specific infections, such as candidiasis or yeast infection. The mushrooms listed below are powerful immune boosters, but they can also be used to strengthen the body's fight against cancer. (See Chapter Six for more information on these mushrooms.)

Echinacea *(Echinacea angustifolia; purpurea)*

Despite a divided scientific community, I believe that echinacea is a highly effective, broad-spectrum antibiotic and immune booster. Echinacea kills bacteria, fungus, and viruses. At the same time, it boosts immune function. Studies have shown that echinacea increases production of interleukins, tumor necrosis factor, and CD4 cells. It is also anti-inflammatory and works wonderfully against colds, flu, and all forms of infection, including yeast infection. When combined with saw palmetto, it is effective in the treatment of prostatitis (inflammatory swelling of the prostate usually due to a bacterial infection).

Take echinacea Monday, Tuesday, Thursday, and Friday, with Wednesdays and weekends off. Do not take while pregnant. Be sure to tell your physician if you are taking Echinacea for anything, including HIV, as it interacts with certain medications. Take as directed, in tincture, tablet, or tea form.

Goldenseal *(Hydrastis canadensis; Ranunculaceae)*

Goldenseal can be taken in tea, tablet, or tincture form or applied topically. As a tea, boil one or two tablespoons of the dried herb in two cups of water. Let steep for twenty minutes before drinking. As a tincture, take thirty drops, in water or apple juice, up to three times per day. Goldenseal reduces inflammation; stimulates the liver to cleanse the blood; promotes improved digestion; treats fungal, viral, and bacterial infections; regulates menstrual cycles; reduces irritation from hemorrhoids; is effective against *Candida albicans* overgrowth; and treats the skin eruptions and rashes that occur with candidiasis. Goldenseal is also effective against the symptoms of flu and lowers fever. Don't use for longer than two weeks because it can irritate the urinary or digestive tract. Frequency: WWO.

Uña de Gato (Cat's Claw; *Uncaria tometosa*)

This Peruvian herb is antibacterial, anti-inflammatory, antiviral, and immune boosting. It has been used for thousands of years by Native American healers to treat infections; digestive disorders; inflammatory disorders, such as arthritis and bursitis; genital herpes and herpes zoster; allergies; ulcers; menstrual irregularities and PMS; candidiasis; and asthma. Uña de Gato has long been used by South American healers in the treatment of cancer, which has brought it to the attention of scientists and physicians, many of whom have reported remarkable anecdotal cases in which the herb has been used to successfully treat several types of cancer, including breast cancer. Look for Uña de Gato that is marked "prima" and is free of TOAs (tetracyclic oxindole alkaloids, chemical antagonists that can greatly inhibit Uña de Gato's positive effects).

Maitake Mushroom Extract

This is a wonderful immune booster and offers protection against cancer. Choose NOW brand Beta Maitake or Maitake Gold by MegaFood and F Frequency: WWO. (See Chapter Seven for more information on maitake mushrooms.)

Mushroom Extract

Choose Stamets 7 by Eclectic Institute. This is a highly potent mixture of seven mushroom extracts, including maitake, shiitake, reishi, and enoki. (See Chapter Seven for more on each of these mushrooms.) Another excellent mixture is MegaFood's Maitake Gold. Frequency: WWO.

Turmeric *(Curcuma longa)*

A staple in Indian cooking and Ayurvedic medicine, turmeric is anti-inflammatory and inhibits platelet aggregation. Research has shown that curcumin, a compound found in turmeric, prevents the development of cancer in animals that have been exposed to powerful carcinogens. Turmeric may disrupt a chemical chain of events that would otherwise lead to malignancy, according to work done at the M.D. Anderson Cancer Center in Houston. Frequency: WWO. Notify your doctor, as it can interact with therapies.

Cumin *(Cuminum cyminum)*

Cumin may inhibit platelet aggregation and prevent urinary tract cancers. Scientists in Israel found that men who eat cumin regularly experience lower rates of cancers of the bladder and prostate. Indian scientists confirmed these findings. They also found that cumin triggers production of a detoxifying enzyme, called GST (glutathione transferase), which is known to have strong cancer-inhibiting properties. Be sure to notify your healthcare provider if you take this herb. Frequency: WWO.

Pau d'Arco

Derived from the bark of a tall, flowering tree in Brazil *(Tabebuia avellanedae, T. impetiginosa)*, pau d'arco is taken most often as a tea, extract, or in capsules, all of which are widely available in most natural foods stores. Pau d'arco has powerful antibacterial, antiviral, and anti-inflammatory properties. The extract can be applied topically for bites and stings, infections, and inflammations. It is available as dried, shredded bark or in capsules and liquid extract (often standardized for lapachol content). Frequency: WWO.

Prostate Health

The following herbs and supplements are highly effective in the treatment of benign prostate hyperplasia (or hypertrophy), as well as prostatitis, the swelling of the prostate due to infection.

Pygeum *(Pygeum africanum)*

This herb is harvested from an evergreen tree native to Africa and widely used in Europe to treat benign prostate hyperplasia (BPH). One study showed that 80 percent of subjects taking pygeum had significant improvement in urine flow and other symptoms related to BPH. Pygeum is widely available in natural foods stores and pharmacies. Standard dosage is one hundred milligrams. Take as directed, but after one month, reduce to five days a week, or WWO.

Saw Palmetto *(Serenoa repens)*

Saw palmetto is used to treat swelling or enlargement of the prostate, but it also blocks the very process that leads to prostate cancer. The prostate becomes enlarged when the male testosterone is converted into dihydrotestosterone. Testosterone, which is essential for muscle development, libido, and many male physical characteristics, is not the cause of prostate disorders. Rather it is the conversion of the hormone into dihydrotestosterone, which is accomplished by the production of the enzyme 5-alphareductase. Saw palmetto inhibits that enzyme's actions and stops the conversion of testosterone into the troubling metabolite. It is this very process that also leads to cancer of the prostate.

Remarkably, saw palmetto relieves the symptoms of enlarged prostate, often very quickly, and without side effects if used in combination and is of high quality.

The June 17, 1995 issue of *The Lancet* (345:1529) reported that a compound in saw palmetto called B-sitosterol significantly reduced prostate symptoms. Two groups of men, both suffering from symptoms of prostate enlargement, or benign prostatic hyperplasia (BPH), were compared. One group received twenty milligrams of beta-sitosterol three times a day; the other got a placebo, or a non-therapeutic sugar pill. Flow rates were significantly improved in the men who were given the saw palmetto compound. No change was observed in those taking the sugar pill.

Saw palmetto has actually been shown to work better than the most commonly used drugs on the market for BPH, and with no significant side effects.

Saw palmetto is widely available in natural foods stores and pharmacies. Take as directed. Purchase brands that contain 85 to 95 percent fatty acids and sterols, which are the active ingredients of the herb.

Zinc

The prostate uses more zinc than any other organ in the body. Zinc boosts immune function and supports prostate health. Take fifteen to thirty milligrams, five days a week, or WWO, as daily use may increase prostate size.

Combine saw palmetto, echinacea, and zinc to treat prostatitis and BPH.

Combine pygeum, saw palmetto, lycopene, zinc, essential fatty acids, and pumpkinseed extract. These substances combine well to treat prostate problems.

Activated Quercetin

This powerful antioxidant has been show to relieve prostate swelling. It is also good for hay fever and colds. For prostatitis, take six hundred milligrams per day, WWO.

Prostamino Plus by MegaFood, Prostate Defense by North Star Nutritionals, and Gaia Prostate Liquid Phyto-Caps

These formulas combines many of the herbs and supplements already mentioned to promote prostate health.

Heart Disease

Be sure to see your doctor or healthcare provider for the treatment of heart disease or for any symptom that might suggest the presence of heart disease.

The following supplements and herbs have been shown to promote healthy heart function. Some lower cholesterol; others increase HDL (good) cholesterol; still others strengthen the heart itself. Always remember that when it comes to heart disease, diet is the first and most important self-help treatment tool. The following herbs and supplements can support a healthy diet and the medical treatments that your doctor prescribes.

Coenzyme Q10

This natural antioxidant is widely available in natural food stores. A three-year Australian study found that when patients who underwent coronary bypass surgery were given daily supplements of coenzyme Q10, their hearts recovered more quickly, the pumping strength of the heart improved, and their hearts tolerated more stress. All of these indicators far surpassed a control group who had also undergone bypass surgery, but were given placebo after the operation. Other research has suggested that CoQ10, as it is frequently called, improves energy production of the heart cells and may reduce the symptoms associated with congestive heart failure. I always recommend a high absorption CoQ10 when my patients take a statin (like Lipitor, Vytorin, Simvastatin, or Crestor) or have a cardiomyopathy. Common dosages range from sixty to two hundred milligrams per day in soft gel capsules. An excellent CoQ10 product is Carni Q-Gel Forte with L-carnitine or the most recent stabilized ubiquinol form called Super Bio Active CoQ10 available at www.LEF.org. Take the sixty-milligram dose, one to three capsules per day or just fifty milligrams once per day of the Bio Active form. These are highly absorbable forms of CoQ10. Remember WWO, Wednesday and the weekends off.

Hawthorne (Crataegus oxyacantha)

This herb, derived from the leaves and berries of a spiny tree native to Europe, is now being used widely in the treatment of heart disease. The rich supply of flavonoids in Hawthorne reduces the contraction of blood vessels and, in the process, lowers blood pressure. (*Japanese Journal of Pharmacology,* 43:242, 1987.) Hawthorne has also been shown to strengthen the contracting force of the heart muscle, reduce arrhythmias, and may help in the treatment of heart failure (*Fortschr Medical Journal:* 20–21, 1993). Hawthorne also lowers cholesterol, and animal studies have shown that it reverses atherosclerosis. (*Biochem Pharm:* 33:3491, 1984.) Hawthorne may also reduce the severity of angina, or chest pain, and has been shown to lower the risk of death in people with proven heart disease. (*Lancet:* 342:1007, 1993; *Journal of Traditional Chinese Medicine* 4:293, 1984.) Hawthorne comes in capsules or as a tincture (drops). Take as directed— usually one hundred to two hundred milligrams, or about fifteen drops, three times per day, twenty minutes before meals, for thirty days. No adverse side effects have been reported.

Soluble Fiber

Three grams per day of water-soluble fiber, such as that from barley, oat, rice bran, or beans, have been shown to lower blood cholesterol, according to a study published in the *Journal of the American Medical Association.* Soluble fiber has been shown to lower LDL cholesterol levels by 10 to 15 percent and total cholesterol by 3 to 6 percent. Eat at least three servings of fiber-rich foods each day.

Psyllium Husks and Seeds

This is a common ingredient in laxatives and digestive medicines, such as Metamucil. It works like oat bran, with similar side effects. Psyllium may be purchased in pharmacies without a prescription. Take one teaspoon mixed with water four times a week (WWO) as a fiber additive until you have a 90 percent whole food, high-fiber diet (Liv-it).

Gugulipid

Extracts from this natural plant herb can lower cholesterol by 21 percent and triglycerides by 25 percent. At the same time, it can raise HDL (the good cholesterol) by 60 percent—all in just three to eight weeks, researchers have shown. It also changes Pattern B small dense LDL particles (not good) to large buoyant LDL (good) particles. Gugulipid is widely available in natural and health food stores. No adverse effects on the liver, blood sugar, or other blood factors have been reported. Take up to five hundred milligrams of a standardized preparation, three times per day, on Monday, Tuesday, Thursday, and Friday (WWO).

Garlic

Garlic protects blood fats and cholesterol in the blood from being oxidized by free radicals, thus preventing the first step in atherosclerosis, or cholesterol plaques. Garlic may also lower cholesterol and prevent platelets from coagulating and forming blood clots in the arteries; it is an anticoagulant. Eat up to one clove per day, four times a week (WWO). You can also take garlic powder and Kyolic, an unscented form of garlic in capsules. If you undergo surgery, you must stop garlic one week prior because it can increase surgical bleeding.

Vitamin C

Vitamin C lowers cholesterol and prevents oxidation of fats and cholesterol in the arteries, thus preventing atherosclerosis. Take five hundred to one thousand milligrams per day, four days a week (WWO).

Vitamin E

Be sure to choose a vitamin E supplement that contains all four tocopherols and all four tocotrienols. Researchers found that one hundred to two hundred International Units (IU) significantly reduced the risk of sudden death from heart attacks in both men and women. Men who took vitamin E supplements for at least two years experienced 37 percent fewer heart attacks, when compared to men who took a placebo. Women who took vitamin E experienced a 41 percent reduction in heart attacks. One sixteen-nation analysis showed that cholesterol and vitamin E levels were the clearest predictors of heart attacks in middle-aged men. However, there has been recent debate about whether vitamin E is helpful or not. Vitamin E can lower cholesterol up to 15 percent and LDL cholesterol eight percent within four weeks. For patients with extremely highly cholesterol levels—greater than three hundred milligrams per deciliter—the drop in cholesterol was 31 percent in four weeks. Take four hundred IU per day, four days per week (WWO).

Researchers from Brigham's and Women's Hospital in Boston found that five hundred milligrams of vitamin C and four hundred IU of vitamin E slowed progression of atherosclerosis in patients who had recently undergone bypass surgery.

Pantethine

Take three hundred milligrams three times per day for thirty days and then twice a day, four days per week (WWO).

Important note: All of these supplements should not be taken at once. Please consult your doctor or healthcare provider for guidance.

Improved Digestion

The following substances restore healthy intestinal flora, will improve digestion, and help alleviate dyspepsia.

Megazymes by MegaFood

This supplement enhances digestion, promotes healthy intestinal function and elimination, improves symptoms related to colitis and irritable bowel, and helps prevent cancer. New York City cancer specialist Nicholas Gonzalez, MD, uses digestive enzymes as a cornerstone of his cancer program. It must be introduced slowly, under medical guidance.

PB 8 by Nutrition Now

This probiotic formula contains soil-based organisms, including lactobacillus. It assists in repopulating the bowel with friendly bacteria; it's particularly useful during dietary changes, when on antibiotics, or as a treatment for gas, irritable bowel, enteritis, or colitis.

MegaFlora by MegaFood

This supplement is a big help when you are constipated. Soaking beans with two opened capsules of MegaFlora, which contains *Lactobacillus casei*, will mitigate the beans' gas-causing properties.

Activated Charcoal

Helps reduce chronic gas.

Peppermint Plus by Enzymatic Therapy

This supplement is helpful for indigestion or excess gas.

Headaches

The following substances may help those who suffer from occasional or chronic headaches, as well as migraines.

Feverfew

Feverfew is a dried herb that is widely available in capsules and tinctures. Take as directed.

Magnesium Caps by Country Life

Magnesium relieves headaches, including migraines; promotes healthy bowel function, especially for people who suffer from constipation; and calms heart irregularities. Please note that people with diminished kidney function must be supervised by a doctor and undergo blood tests to determine if magnesium therapy is safe for them.

Allergies, Asthma, Nasal Congestion, and Colds

Similasan Brand Nasal Spray

Use Similasan in place of Rhinocort or Flonase nasal sprays. While not as effective as steroids, these are safer and frequently are enough to get the job done.

NutriBiotic Nasal Spray

This natural product is both a decongestant and an antibiotic.

Magnesium

Take one to two magnesium capsules per day (see above information about safe use).

Bones, Joints, and Arthritis

Uña de Gato

Take this herb for arthritis and immune stimulation. (See the previous chapter for a larger discussion about uña de gato).

Devil's Claw

This herb is used primarily in the treatment of arthritic pain. May also be used as a cleanser of the lymph system. Analgesic properties compare in strength to cortisone or Indocin. Do not use during pregnancy.

Turmeric (curcumin extract)

Turmeric is a potent antioxidant and liver protector.

Joint Factors by Nature's Purest or Lifewise

These are formulas designed to maintain joint health.

MSM by Lifewise or NOW

Take three thousand to twelve thousand milligrams per day to aid tissue healing and for any variety of arthritis. It is sold in powder form, which can be added to tea or applesauce, or in nine hundred or thousand-milligram capsules.

Artho-7 by Gero Vital

This supplement is used to treat arthritis.

Liprinol by Prevail

This extract of the green-lipped mussel from New Zealand is used to treat arthritis. Provides pain relief and tissue repair.

Bone Formula by MegaFood

Take as a supplement to prevent and treat osteoporosis. It helps to rebuild bone. Take full dose for thirty days and then two to four tablets a day, four days per week (WWO).

Joint Advantage from Dr. David Williams

This formula is designed to build stronger, healthier joints.

OsteoGuard and Osteoking

Used to heal fractures or to treat osteoporosis.

Vitamin K2, Strontium, and Potassium Citrate

These supplements are useful in the treatment of osteoporosis.

Mind, Memory, and Emotional Support

The following substances support mental clarity, memory, and emotional stability.

Ginkgo Biloba

A powerful antioxidant, ginkgo biloba has been used traditionally to promote circulation throughout the body, especially to the brain and heart. It has been shown to help reduce dizziness, migraine headaches, and tinnitus, or ringing in the ears. Available in pill form. Use as directed at first, and then take four days per week (WWO).

Neuromins DHA (two hundred milligrams)

This vegetarian omega-3 fatty acid is prevalent in the brain and helps to improve mental function. This supplement, in combination with ginkgo biloba and DMAE, greatly improves memory. Take four days per week (WWO).

Kava Kava by Nature's Purest

This herb acts as a natural version of valium. Take four days per week (WWO).

St. John's Wort Supreme by Gaia

This herb is a very effective natural antidepressant. Take it as an alternative to Celexa, Lexapro, Prozac, Zoloft, or Luvox. Take four days per week (WWO).

Vinpocetine

This supplement enhances mental function.

Magnesium

Take one to two magnesium capsules per day (see above information about safe use).

Support for the Liver

Milk Thistle *(Silybum Marianum)*

A very effective herb for rebuilding and healing the liver. It is also a powerful antioxidant. Researchers at Case Western Reserve University in Cleveland have shown that the active ingredient in milk thistle, silymarin, promotes the recovery of the liver. They also found that it protects mice against skin cancer. Milk thistle is available as a dried herb—it is boiled in water and used as a tea—or in drops, capsules, or tinctures. Take four days per week (WWO).

Andrographis Paniculata by Planetary Formulas

This is another liver protector and potent immune stimulator.

When used wisely and with restraint, supplements and herbs can provide a great boost to your body's healing powers. They can address specific illnesses—usually with few, if any, harmful side effects—while they promote your own healing abilities. It is wise to seek competent guidance in the use of supplements and herbs, especially if you use more than one at a time.

CHAPTER EIGHT

Exercise: A Little Will Change Your Life

When Andrea first came to see me in 1996, she was suffering from panic attacks and a weak heart. I ran a series of tests on her, including an ejection fraction, which measures how much blood is being expelled from the heart's left ventricle with every contraction. An ejection fraction of fifty-five, which is the minimum normal, means that 55 percent of the blood in that chamber is being pumped out of the chamber with each contraction of the heart. Anything below 50 percent is abnormal (normal is 55 to 75 percent) and means that only half the blood in the left ventricle is being pumped out with each beat. Such an ejection fraction indicates that the heart is in a weakened state and is significantly diseased.

Upon my first series of tests, I found that Andrea's ejection fraction was 25 percent. Other tests confirmed that she was suffering from severe cardiomyopathy, or the weakening and atrophy of the heart muscle. She was very close to suffering heart failure. In fact, she already had a close call and nearly died of heart failure. She was only thirty-six years old.

In addition to these problems, Andrea was about twenty pounds overweight and suffered from an array of allergies and chronic fatigue, a consequence of her weakened heart and overall poor health.

I changed her diet dramatically, switching her to a whole-foods GVB Liv-it, based largely on whole grains, especially quinoa, barley, and brown rice; lots of beans; vegetables; and a type of seaweed called *nori,* which is loaded with minerals and antioxidants. Andrea, who was born in Jamaica, had been used to eating certain grains and beans as a child but had adopted much of the American way of eating when she moved to the United States in her youth. I allowed her to eat fish every week but eliminated all dairy products, red meat, and processed foods.

In addition, I put her on an exercise routine that consisted of daily walking. With her heart in such jeopardy, I was careful to limit her speed and the distance she walked, insisting initially that she walk in ten-minute sessions. It didn't matter to me how far she walked. I just wanted her to exercise. I knew that as long as her diet was healthy, even a little bit of walking would improve the strength of her heart. I also put her on a multivitamin; a magnesium supplement; an herb called hawthorne berry, which strengthens the heart; and the antioxidant Coenzyme Q10 to improve the strength of her heart. Conventional Western medicines were also used. For now, the supplement arginine was stopped.

After three months, Andrea started to show real signs of improvement. Her energy levels increased significantly, and her heart ejection fraction was also getting higher. At that point, I took her off of the hawthorne berry and the magnesium supplement—the latter was no longer necessary because her diet was providing her with all the magnesium she needed. I also increased her walking distance and began to add a small amount of resistance training to her program in the form of hand-held weights. Western medicines were likewise reduced.

After ten months, Andrea's ejection fraction had reached fifty-five and was safely in the normal range. Today, she has lost weight, suffers no more panic attacks or allergies, and walks three miles a day. She has no signs of cardiomyopathy or any other form of heart disease.

"I am amazed at the progress I have made," Andrea said recently. "I had seen so many doctors before, and no one could figure out what to do for my heart and other problems. This approach changed my life."

When it comes to improving your health, no other immune booster affects your life as dramatically as exercise. Exercise boosts immune function, lowers blood pressure, improves cardiovascular health and fitness, raises levels of HDL (the good cholesterol), reduces weight, elevates mood, improves mental health, and protects against many forms of cancer.

Even more important, perhaps, is that exercise strengthens your willpower and gives you a sense that you can overcome virtually any problem. Numerous studies have shown that those who exercise are more likely to maintain a healthy diet than those who do not exercise. Why? Because their systems are cleaned on a regular basis. In addition, I believe that exercise strengthens willpower, so exercisers are less likely to indulge in unhealthy foods. In any case, there is nothing in any pill or potion that will change your life as much as regular exercise will.

First, a Warning

Before you start exercising, it's essential to do two things: change your diet to lower your fat intake and protect your heart; and see your healthcare provider for a complete exam and possibly a stress test.

I remember a story about Nathan Pritikin, the famed diet and health advocate who saved the lives of tens of thousands of people with his "80:10:10" (carbohydrate/fat/protein), low-fat, low-cholesterol diet and gentle exercise program. He repeatedly warned people in his writings to change their diets before they did any sort of demanding physical activity, because he feared that if people didn't lower their cholesterol levels and take the stress off their hearts, they would substantially raise their risk of having a heart attack.

One day, Nathan received a call from running advocate Jim Fixx, author of *The Complete Book of Running,* who railed against Pritikin for scaring people away from running. "Don't you know that you are keeping people from changing their lives for the better?" Fixx said to Pritikin.

"What's your blood cholesterol level?" Pritikin asked Fixx.

Fixx told Pritikin that it was in the high two hundreds. Pritikin replied that if Fixx didn't change his own diet, he would die of a heart attack. Fixx scoffed at Pritikin and flatly told him to stop scaring people.

It wasn't long after that conversation that Fixx did indeed die of a heart attack while running. Don't do the same thing.

The exercise program I describe in Chapter Twelve is a very gentle, non-strenuous program. The first part of my three-part exercise program is walking. However, I regard exercise without dietary change as dangerous.

The second step is to heed your healthcare provider's advice on exercise, especially until your cholesterol level falls into the healthy ranges (less than 150 for most of us; less than 130 in diabetics and those with heart or kidney disease).

Life Extension

Perhaps for all of these reasons, exercise is also associated with longer life. Numerous studies have shown that those who exercise regularly live longer and have lower rates of illness. And you don't have to be consumed by exercise in order to enjoy all of these benefits.

A study published in the *Journal of the American Medical Association* divided a population of 13,344 men and women into five groups, each one rated according to the members' physical fitness and the regularity and intensity with which they exercised.

Group One was composed of sedentary people who did no exercise at all. Group Two was made up of people who walked for thirty minutes a day, three or four days per week. The people in Group Three exercised regularly; Group Four was composed of athletes; Group Five, marathon runners and others who exercised intensely.

As you might expect, the people in Group One died the soonest and in the greatest numbers. What surprised the researchers at the Cooper Clinic in Dallas, Texas, however, was that the greatest improvement in life span and overall health was obtained by Group Two. Simply walking a half hour a day cut the group's chances of having a heart attack or cancer in half. The other three groups enjoyed only slightly better health benefits than those of group two. Moderation may have been the real marker.

Cancer rates differed dramatically among the five groups. When comparing cancer rates among the men, the researchers found that the men who did not exercise had four times more cancer than those who were physically fit. Of the women, those who did not exercise had sixteen times the cancer rate than those who were physically active.

Other research has confirmed these findings. A study published in the *New England Journal of Medicine* (February 25, 1993) found that men between the ages of forty-five and fifty-four who take up a vigorous sport live, on average, ten months longer than those who remain sedentary. I think they'd live a lot longer if they also ate according to the Food Mantra: fresh, whole and unprocessed organic fiber (grains, vegetables, beans, fruit, nuts, and seeds).

It is well known that exercise improves cardiovascular health and lowers the risk of heart attack and stroke.

A leisurely stroll at a pace of three miles per hour can significantly reduce a woman's risk of suffering from heart disease, according to a study published in the *Journal of the American Medical Association* (December 18, 1991). The researchers divided a group of women into four groups, with three of them walking at different speeds. One group did a twenty-minute mile; another a fifteen-minute mile; and a third did a twelve-minute mile. The fourth group did not walk at all and served as a control group.

All of the walkers experienced a 6 percent increase in their HDL cholesterol levels, no matter what speed they walked. Yes, the faster-paced walkers had greater levels of fitness, but their HDL levels were the same as those who strolled.

Such an increase in HDL levels can have a profound impact on the risk of heart disease. "That increase in HDL translates into an 18 percent drop in heart disease risk," said the study's lead author, John J. Duncan, PhD, of the Cooper Institute for Aerobics Research.

And that's purely from taking a stroll a few times per week.

One of the more underappreciated effects of exercise is that it tends to dramatically affect your food choices. People who regularly exercise tend to consume more complex carbohydrates, those that come from whole grains, vegetables, beans, and fruits, according to a 1994 study published in the *American Journal of Clinical Nutrition* (59:728S–734S). In addition, those who exercise regularly eat less fat than those who maintain a sedentary lifestyle, according to a study published in the *American Journal of Public Health* (1995; 85: 240–244). Little wonder, therefore, that the big difference between those who lose weight and keep it off versus those who adopt a weight loss program but regain the weight they may have lost is regular exercise.

While exercise has an independent effect on health, it also promotes healthier habits in other areas of your life. That greasy cheeseburger, with the fat dripping off of it, is a lot less appealing after you've had a vigorous workout or just walked a mile and you feel really clean and healthy inside.

Exercise and Immune Response

One independent benefit from exercise is immune boosting. When it comes to the effects of exercise on the immune system, moderation is the key. As long as you don't overdo your workout, exercise can have a profound effect on your immune system. Among the many strengthening effects of exercise are the following:

- It increases the number and aggressiveness of macrophages; with regular exercise, macrophages are far more effective at destroying bacteria, viruses, and cancer cells.
- It stimulates macrophages to produce more cytokines, including tumor necrosis factor, which destroys cancer cells and tumors.
- It triggers granulocytes to become more active against infection, including those of the skin.
- It makes natural killer (NK) cells more aggressive against cancer cells and tumors. Even the elderly show stronger natural killer cell activity when they take up an exercise program.

These findings may tell us why men and women who regularly exercise have lower rates of the common cancers, including those of the breast, colon, and prostate. Exercise also appears to offer women significant protection against breast cancer.

One study, done jointly by the National Cancer Institute and Shanghai Cancer Institute in China, showed that women whose jobs are sedentary, who consequently expend very little energy each day, have a breast cancer rate that is 30 percent above the average. On the other hand, women whose jobs require them to be very active and burn a lot of calories each day, have breast cancer rates that are 10 and 20 percent below the average.

Another study showed that women who exercised an average of forty-eight minutes a week—less than one hour—were significantly less likely to develop breast cancer than those who did not exercise at all. Those women who exercised about four hours weekly had the lowest rates of breast cancer.

Those who were physically active had 25 to 50 percent fewer cases of cancer than those who lived sedentary lifestyles.

Physical activity in youth appears to be particularly important, especially for women. Dr. Rose Frisch of the Harvard School of Public Health studied a group of 5,400 women. Dr. Frisch found that those women who, during their college years, exercised regularly or participated in athletics had half the rate of breast cancer later in life than those who did not exercise or participate in athletics during college.

Balance Is the Key

Few immune boosters and health promoters demonstrate the need for balance better than exercise. Too much exercise is nearly as bad as too little: Excessive strenuous exercise depresses the immune system. During the last twenty years, we have seen this point demonstrated all too persuasively, as numerous highly trained athletes have been struck down with cancer.

Highly (over)trained athletes often have higher rates of infection, as well. Studies that compared the immune responses of highly conditioned athletes to those of the average people have found that the athletes have more infections and weaker immune systems. The number and aggressiveness of lymphocytes, blood and saliva levels of immunoglobulins, and the ratio of CD4 to CD8 cells was lower in athletes than average people. Natural killer cell activity was also lower in the highly conditioned athletes.

The physical and mental stresses associated with high levels of athletic competition appear to weaken immunity. These levels of stress are also associated with extraordinary losses of antioxidants. A study done on the German National Field Hockey team just before the 1988 Olympic games found that the intense exercise and psychological stresses left the athletes in a weakened immune state. Some of the players had CD4 counts similar to those found in AIDS patients.

Remarkably, studies have shown that a nutritious diet, coupled with antioxidant supplementation, restores immune function. One study showed that marathon runners who were given vitamin C after a race had lower rates of respiratory infections than those who were not given the vitamin C.

A Powerful Mood Booster

Exercise elevates mood, creates feelings of well-being, confidence, and even euphoria. These effects occur in part because of the increased production of endorphins by the brain during exercise. Endorphins are opium-like compounds that the brain produces after about ten to twenty minutes of steady exercise, including simple walking. Exercise can also significantly improve mental health.

As far back as 1990, a study published in *Postgraduate Medicine* (July 1990) reported that people who had formerly suffered from depression and other emotional problems experienced reductions in stress and anxiety, and had fewer bouts of depression after they began exercising. Their capacity to deal with stress also increased with regular exercise. When stressful situations arose, they did not succumb to self-criticism and other kinds of negative thinking. The researchers also found that consistent exercise seemed to bring about a type of emotional transformation among those who maintained an exercise program consistently. The people who participated in the study reported feeling healthier, emotionally brighter, and far more positive about life than before they began exercising. Even depression has been relieved by consistent exercise. In fact, exercise has been shown to be as effective as medication in the treatment of depression.

When it comes to relieving stress and boosting mood, aerobic exercise seems to have a greater impact than anaerobic exercises, such as weight training. When the psychological effects of aerobic exercise were compared with weight training and no exercise at all, researchers found that aerobic exercise had the most elevating effects on mood and well-being. But weight training is better at efficiently reducing percent body fat. My advice: do both!

How Much Exercise Do You Need?

One of the most authoritative groups of fitness experts, the American College of Sports Medicine (ACSM), recommends that people who are not exercising currently but want to start an exercise program should start out with thirty minutes of "moderately intense" physical activity most days of the week. Thirty minutes of walking, four to six days per week, meets those criteria.

Most important, the ACSM states that those thirty minutes per day of exercise can be cumulative, meaning that you can do three sessions of ten minutes each and still derive tremendous benefit. That means that if you walk ten minutes in the morning, ten minutes at lunch, and ten minutes more after dinner, you've got your thirty minutes in.

As I stated earlier, walking does not have to be at an accelerated pace. Even a ten-minute stroll provides tremendous benefit. As your fit-ness increases, pick up the pace and lengthen the distance. If you use a tread-mill, begin at 3 percent elevation and gradually work up to 10 percent. Try waving your outstretched arms as you walk.

In addition to walking, I recommend a small amount of weight, or resistance, training. Resistance training improves strength, endurance, and bone density. It is especially important for women concerned with osteo-porosis, because it accelerates bone breakdown and rebuilding, thus making bones stronger and more flexible over time. Resistance training also raises HDL levels, makes muscles bigger, cushions the body against falls, increases range of motion and mobility, and creates stronger stomach, back, leg, and hamstring muscles.

Resistance training exercises can be done once or twice per week. They break down muscles, encouraging the body to rebuild larger, stronger mus-cles with greater endurance. But muscle rebuilding takes time, so you should allow at least three days between weight training sessions.

Some of the best resistance training exercises are the simple old-fashioned kind: sit-ups, push-ups, and knee-bends. You can start out doing as many repetitions of each as you are able to. That may mean five sit-ups, five push-ups, and five knee-bends. If five is too many, do fewer and work up to five. Then work your way up to ten, and then fifteen, and so on. You will see your fitness improving fairly rapidly if you are consistent.

Resistance training also involves weights. The most effective of these are small dumbbells and ankle weights that strap onto your ankles and are used to strengthen your legs. I prefer ten-pound and fifteen-pound Cap brand dumbbells.

It's very important that when you begin the exercise program I have outlined in Chapter Eleven, you do it in a way that is enjoyable for you, not in a way that causes you pain or suffering, which will only result in injury or worse. Start slowly and gently, and give yourself time to develop better fitness. If you adopt the program that I have outlined, you will see rapid improvements in your endurance, strength, and energy levels. And you'll have a good time doing it.

CHAPTER NINE

Balance, Beliefs, and Stress: Humor Helps

Sometimes the healthiest things we can do are to lighten up and get a little silly. Laughter can be medicinal, and even a little smile can make you feel better. Here are a few jokes I've enjoyed:

One day a patient said to his doctor, "Doc, are you sure I'm suffering from pneumonia? I read about one patient who was diagnosed with pneumonia and died of typhus."

"Don't worry," said the doctor. "If I treat a patient with pneumonia, he will die of pneumonia."

A surgeon woke his patient after an operation and said, "I'm going to have to operate on you again because I left my rubber gloves inside of you."

The patient replied, "Just charge me for the gloves and leave me alone."

A patient said to her doctor, "I want to die like my grandmother, who died peacefully in her sleep. Not screaming like all the passengers in her car."

Here's some medical advice that parents will understand: if you have a tension headache, do what it says on the aspirin bottle—"Take two aspirin" and "Keep away from children."

Three elderly sisters lived in the same house. One was running a bath one day, put her foot into the tub and asked, "Am I getting into the tub or out?" Another stopped on the stairs for a moment and wondered out loud, "Am I going up or down?" A third sister heard the confusion of the other two and said to herself, "Knock on wood, I'm glad I don't have those problems." With that, she tapped her knuckles on a nearby table. She then yelled up to her two sisters, "I'll be up to help you both, as soon as I answer the door."

We live in a cynical age in which modern social pressures encourage us to adopt a pessimistic and negative approach to life. What such cultural trends deny is the overwhelming forces of evolution, which have encouraged humans to be optimistic about the future (optimism makes us more resourceful and better able to survive); more social (people are more likely to survive in groups); and more spiritually oriented (wisdom was cultivated first by those who feared nature, or in traditional terms, God).

These are not mere superficial aspects of our humanity, but deeply imbedded patterns that are held in our genes. Even science has begun to reveal that our very brains are biologically formed to grapple with the notion of a Supreme Creator or Divine Force that animates the universe. We are hardwired with behavior patterns that encourage us to live in close intimacy with one another, to understand ourselves, and, every so often, to see the humor in it all.

Laugh: It Does a Body Good

Laughter creates a wide range of biochemical changes that boost immune function, promote healing, and create pain relief. No doubt you remember the story of Norman Cousins who overcame a painful and life-threatening spinal disease, ankylosing spondylitis, using a variety of mind-body techniques, most notably laughter.

Cousins watched films by Mel Brooks and the Marx Brothers and found that twenty minutes of genuine belly laughter gave him two hours of pain-free sleep. Cousins, who documented his recovery in his now famous book, *Anatomy of an Illness,* referred to laughter as "inner jogging."

Dr. William Fry of Stanford has shown that laughter creates a kind of "jogging" effect on the body and on brain chemistry. Not only does it increase heart rate, muscular activity, respiration, and oxygen exchange, but it also promotes the secretion of endorphins, morphine-like compounds that elevate mood and increase one's sense of well-being and optimism. Endorphins are responsible for what researchers call the "runner's high," or, in the case of laughter, "laugher's high."

Laughter may also promote a stronger immune system, as Norman Cousins' experience suggests. Scientists at Western New England College in Springfield, MA, showed two groups of volunteers very different kinds of films—one group watched Richard Pryor Live, while the other watched educational films. After both groups watched their respective videos, the scientists measured antibody responses to an antigen and found that those who watched Richard Pryor had significantly higher antibody production than those who watched the educational films. Increases in antibodies are linked to lower rates of upper respiratory illness.

The University of California at Berkeley's *Wellness Letter* reported (June 1985) that a study conducted by University of California at Santa Barbara researchers found that laughter was as effective at reducing stress as "more complex biofeedback training programs." As the *Wellness Letter* said, laughter requires no special equipment or training, just a funny bone.

At the Very Least, Put On a Happy Face

There's an old saying: fake it until you make it. That seems like good advice, especially when it's applied to a simple smile.

As it turns out, facial expressions may actually create the associated mood, instead of the other way around. Researchers are finding that a smile increases feelings of happiness, while a frown promotes feelings of sadness or despair—even when nothing in particular makes you happy or sad. The idea that facial expressions affect a person's psychological state was first proposed by Charles Darwin, the British scientist who gave us the theory of evolution. Smiling, Darwin maintained, actually triggers happy emotions, while frowning does the opposite.

Dr. Robert Zajonc, a psychologist at the University of Michigan who has studied the effect of facial expression on brain chemistry, has demonstrated that Darwin's assertion is essentially true, and even has a biochemical basis. Zajonc's theory is based on the fact that facial expressions create very different temperatures in the blood and brain. When you smile, certain muscles in the face tighten and prevent blood from flowing through the cavernous sinus cavity where it is typically warmed. The result is that cooler blood gets to the brain. A frown causes blood to flow through the cavernous sinus, which means that much warmer blood makes its way to the brain.

As it turns out, warm blood and warmer temperatures in the brain trigger chemical changes that promote negative feelings and emotions. Cool temperatures do the opposite: they trigger changes in brain chemistry that promote pleasant feelings and psychological states. By keeping the blood cool, smiling creates the kinds of conditions in the brain that are associated with pleasure and happiness. You might say that a smile mechanically turns on your happy chemicals. By sending warm blood to the brain, a frown does just the opposite. Try out the theory now, for yourself. Put a broad, happy smile on your face, and see if you don't feel better. I do. While this method may not help you overcome genuine grief or deep unhappiness, it's worth using in response to your average, run-of-the-mill funks.

Optimism: Looking on the Bright Side Could Extend Your Life

Positive feelings, no matter how they are derived, are powerful forms of medicine. Optimism is one of the most effective feel-good tools around.

Researchers at the Mayo Clinic in Rochester, Minnesota, reported a fascinating study showing that optimistic people live 19 percent longer than pessimists. In 1962 and 1965, researchers performed extensive personality testing on 839 people in Minnesota County, asking them to explain the causes of life events. The answers determined whether the person fell into one of three groups: optimist, pessimist, or a middle category that had characteristics of both.

The researchers followed the three groups for three decades and found that, overall, optimists had significantly better survival rates than the other two groups, while the pessimists, as a group, had a 19 percent higher death rate.

The study, published in the February 2000 issue of the *Mayo Clinic Proceedings,* found that optimists experienced far less depression and feelings of hopelessness than the other groups. In his editorial in the same issue, Martin Seligman, a psychologist at the University of Pennsylvania, said that pessimism is an identifiable trait, and that it can be changed. (See Chapter Thirteen for information on how you can promote more positive feelings, including optimism.)

A study reported in the British medical journal, *The Lancet* (November 1993), found that people who, early in life, came to believe they are predisposed to life-threatening illnesses actually died sooner than those who did not believe they were predisposed to disease. Researchers followed Chinese-Americans born during certain years, who were believed to be predisposed to lethal diseases. These Chinese-Americans actually died four years sooner, on average, than Chinese-Americans born during other years, and at least four years sooner than Anglo-Americans who, in fact, had the same diseases as the Chinese Americans but had healthier beliefs about the outcomes of those illnesses.

The findings were based on a very large sampling of people—28,169 Chinese Americans and 412,632 Caucasians. Study leader David P. Phillips, PhD, professor of sociology at the University of California, San Diego, suggests that beliefs can have a dramatic effect on health. "Our findings, and those of others, suggest that better mental attitude is associated with better health," said Phillips.

Relaxation, Safety, and Immunity

One of the most powerful tools for promoting optimism and feelings of safety—typically, one enhances the other—is the use of meditation and relaxation techniques. A recent study showed that meditation might have a powerful impact on CD4 cells, even in people who suffer from severe illness.

Scientists at Florida's University of Miami Medical School have found that daily relaxation exercises—that is, the progressive releasing of tension in muscles throughout the body—caused CD4 cells to increase. The study was done on men with HIV, who normally experience a steady decrease in CD4 cells. When Gail Ironson, MD, a psychiatrist at the University of Miami Medical School, and her colleagues followed up with the men a year later, they found that those men who continued to do some form of daily meditation or relaxation exercises were less likely to suffer from AIDS symptoms.

Other research has shown that meditation or relaxation exercises have increased immune cell activity in the face of a disease-causing agent. One study showed an increase in natural killer cells and greater proliferation of lymphocytes in medical school students who practiced a daily relaxation regime.

Charles Alexander, professor of psychology at Maharishi International University in Fairfield, Iowa, and Ellen Langer, a psychologist at Harvard University, have been studying the effects of transcendental meditation on the lifespan of elderly residents in eight Boston-area nursing homes. The researchers found that Transcendental Meditation, commonly referred to as TM, appeared to significantly increase survival rates among nursing home residents whose average age was eighty-one. Three years after the study began; all of those practicing TM were still alive, while 38 percent of the non-meditators at the nursing homes were dead.

Other research has shown that TM appears to lower systolic blood pressure and improves near-point vision, and hearing—all important indicators when determining the rate at which we age. Dr. Jay Glaser, a physician with Marharishi Ayurveda Health Center in Lancaster, Massachusetts, has compared the natural hormone levels DHEA sulfate (S) between meditators and control groups. When maintained at high levels, DHEAS is an indicator of youth and overall good health. People who have meditated ten years or more consistently show strikingly higher levels of DHEAS, in comparison to people of their own age who do not meditate.

Researchers have found that meditation is also a powerful tool for pain relief. Jon Kabat-Zinn, a professor at the University of Massachusetts Medical Center, has used a meditation technique called "mindfulness," the practice of intentionally paying attention to one's breath, one's body, and surroundings, to reduce pain from all kinds of illnesses, including low back pain, heart disease, and cancer.

A kind of mindfulness occurs when we write about our feelings in a diary or journal. This practice creates a closer sense of intimacy with self, greater self-knowledge, and deeper relaxation. It also helps us understand our inner feelings and create deeper states of inner peace. Studies have shown that journal writing can be helpful in controlling stress and boosting immunity. One recent study showed that those who wrote about traumatic or painful events in their lives for four days, twenty minutes a day, increased T cells. (More about this can be found in Chapter Thirteen.)

"There are many forms of relaxation or meditation exercises," said Dr. Ironson. "They can be as simple as muscle relaxation, or meditating on a beautiful place in nature, or repeating a single word (like a mantra) over and over again in your head. We don't have enough data to distinguish the effects of each of these practices on the immune system, but the research so far suggests that all of them—if practiced regularly—seem to have a positive effect."

Deal Effectively with Stress—In All Its Forms

Everyone knows at this point that stress triggers an array of adverse chemical and biological activities. It creates hormonal imbalances, increases LDL cholesterol, and impairs heart, lung, kidney, adrenal, and nervous system function. When it becomes chronic, stress correlates with heart and kidney disease and even premature death. Is it the stress? Is it how stressed individuals react? Or is it both? In 2006, two studies were published showing that anger correlates with reduced lung function and stiffer blood vessels.

Anger is an interesting emotion, because it is often seen as a consequence of stress. In this way, people dismiss their anger, because they use stress as an excuse to be angry. But anger is itself a stressor. Few people realize that at the bottom of anger is fear—the real source of stress.

Often we are angry because we fear that the situation that causes us stress will have a negative outcome. Something important to us is going to turn out badly, we believe, and we are powerless to stop it. This makes us angry. Anger and fear go hand in hand, though we often see them as very different and separate emotional conditions. At the same time, they tend to fuel each other. As things become more stressful (or more fearful), we often become angrier.

Anger and stress give rise to all kinds of destructive behaviors, including drug and alcohol abuse.

Please understand me; I am not saying that anger is entirely bad. On the contrary, I believe that evolution gave us anger to help us recognize when the conditions around us are a threat to our well-being or safety. A crucial lesson in our maturing process, it seems to me, is to learn how to respond appropriately to anger.

This has been borne out by a study conducted by Dr. Sandra P. Thomas, director of The Center for Nursing Research at the University of Tennessee in Knoxville, who studied the effects of anger on women. The study found that repressing feelings of anger, or venting them indiscriminately, could have damaging effects on both health and self-esteem.

Women in poor health, Dr. Thomas found, have a greater tendency to experience anger, but at the same time fail to express it, especially at the person who triggered it. Instead, they reflect on the problem endlessly, ruminating and engaging in internal dialogues that lead to a variety of health problems.

Dr. Thomas found that many physical symptoms arise when a person chronically experiences anger but fails to respond appropriately to it. Among the most common of these physical symptoms are severe headaches, lower backache, shakiness, depression, high blood pressure, excess weight, obesity, and autoimmune disorders, such as arthritis. All of these conditions result, in part, as a consequence of unhealthy reactions to anger. The most common form of unhealthy behavior in the face of anger is keeping it in.

Interestingly, just venting anger at others is not the answer either, Dr. Thomas found. Rage and blaming and attacking others often leads to depression. Dr. Thomas's study showed that depressed women were more likely to experience physical symptoms when angry.

Neither of the two extreme behaviors—repressing anger or venting it willy-nilly—are good strategies for health. Rather, the best approach is to rationally examine the sources of the anger and deal with them effectively.

Dr. Thomas found that the healthiest women spoke to confidants about the problem over which they were angry and then systematically worked through that problem to a reasonable solution. In other words, they recognized that their anger was a legitimate sign of a problem in their environment. They then talked with a confidant about the problem or with the person who stimulated the anger, in such a way as to create a solution to the problem. It is true to a point: "Confession is good for the soul."

Anger that leads to a solution to a problem in one's life is anger that serves a very positive purpose. Solving anger is the key.

The women who used their anger to arrive at solutions experienced the highest levels of self-esteem, Dr. Thomas found.

Just because this research focused on women does not mean that it does not apply to men. Other studies have shown that men who are prone to anger are far more likely to suffer heart attacks than men who are more emotionally calm or balanced.

It's Good to Work and Play Well with Others

Like it or not, we are social beings.

Again, Darwin comes to mind, because we know that humans survived and evolved over hundreds of thousands of years in close communities. Without community, we may have been snuffed out as a species.

Growing up, we all learn very important lessons about community—lessons that we typically think of as ethics or morality. Those honest and capable of love tend to function better in communities than do those who exhibit antisocial behaviors. Indeed, we have learned that antisocial behavior eventually leads to being cast out from the community, a fate that, in ancient times, was tantamount to death. Current science is showing that such lessons are as relevant as ever.

Research has shown that those who have positive connections to their community live longer and enjoy better health, while those who live in isolation are more likely to suffer from illness and die prematurely. One of the best known studies on this is the famed and still perfectly relevant Alameda County study from 1979. Researchers examined the lives of seven thousand residents of Alameda County, California, over a nine-year period. Those residents who were married and had close personal friends and/or church or civic affiliations, lived longer and had fewer illnesses than those who were unmarried or socially isolated. Other studies have repeatedly confirmed these initial findings.

Men, especially, are particularly vulnerable to illness when they live alone, or lose a loved one. Dr. Maradee Davis and her colleagues at the University of California at San Francisco studied 7,651 adults and found that middle-aged men who were unmarried or divorced were twice as likely to die ten years sooner than men who were married or lived with their wives. That finding held true even after accounting for differences in economic situations, smoking habits, drinking, obesity, and physical activity.

"Men who lived alone or with someone other than a spouse had significantly shorter survival times compared with those living with a spouse," Dr. Davis reported in her study, published in the *American Journal of Public Health* (March 1992). The pattern of early death was particularly strong among younger men. "The age-adjusted relative hazard of dying was highest in the youngest age group, forty-five to fifty-four years, and decreased somewhat with increasing age."

Ironically, the same pattern did not exist among women. In an interview with *Natural Health,* Dr. Davis speculated on the reason women fare better than men. "Women have better social support networks, are better at making friends, and seem to take better care of their health than men do," Davis said.

At Duke University Medical School, Redford Williams, Maryland, director of Behavioral Research at Duke, found that those who suffer a heart attack and have no spouse or close personal friend are three times more likely to have a fatal heart attack within five years of the original event than those whose hearts are equally injured but are married or have intimate relationships.

The Duke University research is based on a nine-year follow up study of 1,368 patients who were initially admitted to Duke for cardiac catheterization to diagnose heart disease. "What we found was that those patients with neither a spouse nor a friend were three times more likely to die than those involved in a caring relationship," said Dr. Williams.

For people with both minor and severe heart muscle damage due to a heart attack, the results were consistent. People with heart damage generally faced about a 40 percent chance of dying within five years. Dr. Williams found that those who were married or had a close intimate relationship reduced their risk of suffering a fatal heart attack to 20 percent, while those who lacked intimacy raised their chances of dying to 60 percent.

Other research has consistently supported these findings. Women with breast cancer who participate in a support group live longer than those who try to deal with the disease alone. Scientists are discovering that not only are the recommendations of traditional healers effective, but so too are the guidelines for living offered by spiritual traditions. After reviewing the evidence linking meditation and intimacy to longer life, Dr. Williams said, "It seems evident that the core teachings of most of our religions have been right all along."

A Balanced Life

There seems to be something inherent in us that demands balance in our lives. Workaholism leads to illness, just as chronic weakness, powerlessness, and anger do. When we live too narrow a life—focusing too much on our careers, on ourselves, or on others—we inevitably run into physical and psychological problems.

In Chapter Thirteen, I explore how balance can be found and created in our lives. But for now it's worth asking ourselves, what is this human need for balance? Why is it necessary to learn to give *and* receive? Such speculation inevitably leads from Darwinism to Teleology, the idea that humanity, and the very universe itself, is based on a certain design that makes love or intimate connection essential for health. What we do know is that balance is essential for a long, happy, and fulfilled life. In the end, each person must determine what balance really means for him- or herself and what it looks like in practice.

PART II

The Maximum Healing Program: A Four-Week Program to Boost Your Immune System and Restore Your Health

The Maximum Healing Diet and Lifestyle Program is divided into four parts: diet, exercise, outlook on life, and creating balance in your daily life. What I have written is an invitation to modify your diet and lifestyle, and it represents the ideal changes for you to make. Please be patient with yourself as you transition to healthier habits. These changes can be adopted over time.

CHAPTER TEN

Week One: An Immune-Boosting Diet

A t the foundation of the Maximum Healing Program is a drastically improved way of eating. In this chapter, I offer two separate diets: The Good Health Maintenance Diet and The Maximum Healing Diet. Their names reveal their different purposes.

I designed The Good Health Maintenance Diet specifically for people who are essentially free from symptoms and disease. If you don't have major health problems, but want to boost your immune system, prevent disease, improve your energy, lose some weight, and still enjoy a broad, flexible diet, this is the diet for you.

The Maximum Healing Diet, on the other hand, addresses the needs of those who want to use diet as an effective adjunct for treatment of a serious illness. The Maximum Healing Diet can help you achieve the following health goals:

- Start losing weight immediately
- Significantly boost your immune and cancer-fighting systems
- Reduce your need for oral diabetic medication
- Lower your blood pressure
- Improve your circulation and help you treat claudication
- Reduce and, in many cases, eliminate allergy symptoms
- Reduce and, in some cases, eliminate the pain and other symptoms related to arthritis
- Improve all forms of digestive problems, including constipation, diarrhea, heartburn, and other forms of dyspepsia
- Boost your energy levels

- Improve sleep
- Help you achieve a more youthful vitality and appearance

Here are the two diets, including fourteen days' worth of menus for each regimen.

Diet One: The Good Health Maintenance Diet

Follow this diet if you wish to boost your immune and cancer-fighting systems; lower blood cholesterol; improve digestion; lose weight; increase your intake of vitamins, minerals, and antioxidants, especially vitamin E; increase your energy levels; boost serotonin levels to enhance well-being; and reduce your risk of heart disease, cancer, and other illnesses. If weight loss is one of your goals, keep a food diary of everything you eat for two months.

1. Vegetables: Eat five or more servings of vegetables per day.
2. Fruit: Eat one serving of fruit per day. Cooked berries are preferred if you are overweight.
3. Whole grains: Eat one (cooked) serving per day.
4. Beans: Eat one six- to eight-ounce serving of cooked bean four to five times per week. You may occasionally substitute bean products—including tempeh or tofu and bean-derived sauces like miso, tamari, and shoyu—for whole beans, but these products are highly processed, so their consumption should be limited.
5. Meat: Eat one three-and-a-half-ounce serving (about the size of your palm or a deck of cards) of meat or fish once or twice per week (limit lamb and beef each to once per week and avoid chicken and turkey entirely). If you exercise, you may have up to three servings of meat or fish per week.
6. Eggs: Eat up to two eggs per week. Choose Omega-3 cage-free organic eggs. Eggs can replace fish or red meat. Two eggs equal one fish or red meat serving.
7. Dairy products: Avoid all dairy products, including all forms of milk, cheese, yogurt, and ice cream.

8. Processed foods: Eliminate all processed foods including bread, pastries, rolls, muffins, and all foods containing refined white sugar.

9. Fats: Limit fats to olive, walnut, almond, macadamia nut (macadamia is highest in monounsaturated fats), and sesame oils and small quantities of nut butters, such as almond butter, tahini, and sesame butter.

10. Supplements and herbs: Take one immune-boosting vitamin according to my standard recommendation of WWO (Wednesday and the weekend off) and take supplements and/or herbs designed to address a specific condition that you are battling. (For more information on supplements, see Chapter Seven.)

Diet Two: The Maximum Healing Diet

This diet is designed for maximum immune boosting and cancer fighting; rapid and healthful weight loss; optimal digestion; and maximum energy. Once your health and weight goals have been achieved, you can switch to Diet One: The Good Health Maintenance Diet and enjoy greater flexibility.

1. Breakfast: Eat a warm (not hot) breakfast every day.

2. Vegetables: Eat five to seven servings of vegetables per day.

3. Fruit: Eat at least one serving of fruit daily. If you are overweight, fresh or frozen berries are the best choice.

4. Whole grains: Eat at least two (cooked) servings of whole-grain per day.

5. Beans: Eat one six- to eight-ounce serving of cooked beans or bean products four to five times per week.

6. Bean-derived products: Eat miso or tamari daily as a base for vegetable or noodle soup. (See the recipe section for specific recipes.)

7. Meat: This means free-range animal protein of any type, including fish. You should ask about the fish to find out whether it is farm-raised or wild (preferred). The size of your palm is one serving size. Eggs are a meat, fish, or fowl equivalent. My healthiest patients are vegan.

8. Dairy products: Eliminate all dairy products including milk and cheese (especially if you have breast cysts, lumps, or cancer; painful menses; endometriosis; bunions; an enlarged prostate; or prostate cancer).

9. Tea: Drink black, green, white, or chamomile tea daily. I also recommend using bancha or kukicha twig tea on a daily basis. Both provide only negligible amount of caffeine—so low that you can drink kukicha at night and not have your sleep disrupted. Most people actually feel more relaxed after drinking kukicha tea.

10. Snacks: Eat any of the snacks, nuts (a total of six whole nuts per day, not a handful), seeds, condiments, herbs, and sauces listed below.

11. Desserts: Eat any of the desserts listed in the recipe section of this book.

12. Processed foods: Eliminate all processed foods such as bread, rolls, muffins, and pastries. The only exception is high quality, whole-grain pasta, such as Japanese udon, buckwheat soba, brown rice noodles, and high quality semolina Italian noodles.

13. Fats: Limit to organic extra virgin olive, macadamia, almond, walnut, and sesame oils and small quantities (one to two table-spoons) of nut butters such as almond butter, tahini, and sesame butter.

14. Supplements and herbs: Take a one-a-day vitamin and/or antioxidant formula WWO, plus any herbs and/or supplements that target your specific health issues (see Chapter Seven for additional guidance on the use of supplements and herbs).

Food Guidelines

Whether you choose to follow Diet One or Diet Two, the following guidelines will help you determine which foods to choose from each category and incorporate them into your daily eating plan.

Vegetables

Vegetables are a primary source of nutrition, phytochemicals, and fiber.

- Opt for fresh whenever possible. Frozen vegetables are suitable substitutes when fresh are not available.
- Choose in-season, organic vegetables whenever possible.
- Choose brightly colored vegetables, because they are the richest in nutrition.
- For maximum and rapid weight loss, choose leafy, green, and non-starchy root vegetables, which are extremely low in calories. Avoid starchy vegetables such as potatoes, sweet potatoes, yams, or plantains.
- For maximum satisfaction from low-calorie foods, choose filling vegetables such as winter squash, parsnips, carrots, and collard greens.
- Eat at least one leafy, one round, and one root vegetable per day.
- When in a restaurant, order a salad and two vegetables. Ask that your vegetables be prepared without butter (too much saturated fat). A little olive oil is fine.
- Include one or more of the following "power vegetables" in your diet each day: broccoli, cauliflower, collard greens, freshly roasted and crushed flaxseeds, ginger, onions, kale, mustard greens, mushrooms (shiitake, maitake, reishi, or enoki), or watercress.
- Try sautéing a bunch of collard greens, broccoli, and carrots together in olive oil for ten minutes for three servings of vegetables in a single meal. Or steam kale, carrots, and daikon together for three to seven minutes and, again, you've got three servings of vegetables.
- Make a salad with at least two different vegetables to go along with your dinner each night and you've given yourself two veggie servings.
- Snack on vegetable soup. High-quality organic canned or dehydrated soups are available in most supermarkets. A serving of vegetable soup counts as two or more servings of vegetables.

- If you are at a healthy weight, snack on raw vegetables. (I believe that raw foods stimulate the appetite, so if you are overweight, stick to cooked, soft, and warm vegetables.)

Whole Grains

Whole grains provide the most nearly complete source of nutrition available in the food supply. Highly processed grains, on the other hand, including those found in most cereals, breads, and pastas have been stripped of their vitamins and minerals during processing and are not as rich in nutrition, fiber, and complex carbohydrates.

In addition to being highly nutritious, whole grains are also very filling and satisfying. Once you've mastered their preparation, whole grains can take center stage of your meals, while serving sizes of meats and other proteins are reduced and these foods come to act as flavorful side dishes or condiments.

Please note that if you are overweight (beyond 22 percent body fat for men; 27 percent in women), I recommend that you decrease or eliminate grains from your diet to expedite weight loss. Fill up instead on berries, cooked vegetables and vegetable soups, and beans until you've reached a healthy weight, and then slowly reintroduce grains into your diet, being careful that you don't regain the weight.

Following are the grains I recommend for both diets (see the recipe section for preparation ideas):

Amaranth

Amaranth, a tiny seed-like grain, is rich in calcium, iron, folic acid, and magnesium, and is highest in protein. It has a delicious, earthy flavor and contains no gluten, making it appropriate for those with wheat allergies (Celiac Disease). It is cooked by boiling for fifteen minutes.

Barley

Barley contains soluble fiber, which lowers cholesterol levels, as well as folic acid, magnesium, phosphorus, potassium, and zinc, which make it wonderful for your heart, bones, and immune function. Barley was a staple for the primarily vegetarian gladiators, who were referred to as "barley men"—

as pumped as our modern-day professional wrestlers. In fact the word "burly," meaning big and muscular, is derived from the word "barley."

Barley is lightly refined, or "pearled," and cooks in about an hour. Make a barley stew with vegetables, such as carrots, onions, leeks, and shiitake mushrooms.

Brown Rice

Brown rice is a high-energy food, rich in complex carbohydrates. It's also a good source of B vitamins, such as thiamine and niacin. It provides significant amounts of iron, phosphorus, and magnesium. Unlike many grains, rice contains the amino acid lysine, which makes it a good source of high-quality protein. It contains soluble fiber, which serves to lower blood cholesterol levels. Because of its high complex carbohydrate levels, brown rice increases brain levels of serotonin, the chemical neurotransmitter associated with feelings of well-being, optimism, and the ability to concentrate for long periods of time. Brown rice is available in short, medium, and long grain varieties.

The big difference among the size of the grains is their respective cooking times. Long grain is boiled for about thirty minutes; short grain for about forty minutes. I don't recommend pressure-cooking. Soaking rice overnight prior to cooking cuts cooking time in half.

Buckwheat

Buckwheat, often thought of as a grain but really a grass, is high in calcium.

Millet

Native to Africa and Asia, millet is high in B vitamins, magnesium, copper, and iron. It is often prepared with cauliflower to resemble mashed potatoes (see recipe, page 223).

Oats

Oats provide remarkably high levels of protein, iron, manganese, copper, folic acid, vitamin E, and zinc. They are great for skin, immune function, and digestion.

You can buy oats rolled (instant), steel cut, or whole. Whole oats, which are the least processed, are preferred. Steel cut are my second choice, while rolled are less desirable due to being highly processed. But the more processed oats are, the quicker they cook, so you may want to make your choice based on how much time you have. Whole oats cook in about thirty minutes, steel-cut in about twenty minutes, and rolled in just about six minutes.

Be warned, however, that oats and corn are the grains with the most fat, and as a result they can hinder or stop weight loss, so avoid them if you are overweight.

Quinoa

Quinoa (pronounced keen-wah) is a Peruvian grain that is rich in protein, potassium, riboflavin, magnesium, zinc, copper, manganese, and folic acid. Because it is so nutrient-rich, it is often referred to as a super-grain. Quinoa cooks in about fifteen minutes in boiling water (or just seven minutes if it has been soaked overnight).

Sweet or Glutinous Rice

This highly glutinous form of rice is common in Japan, where it is pounded into dumplings called *mochi*.

Teff

Teff is a tiny, nutrient-packed grain, high in calcium, iron, fiber, protein, and other nutrients. It is also gluten-free, making it a good choice for those with wheat sensitivities. Teff is cooked by boiling in water for fifteen to twenty minutes.

Wheat

Wheat is rich in protein, B vitamins, vitamin E, iron, magnesium, and manganese. Unfortunately, many people are allergic to wheat, and it also has a tendency to cause hypoglycemia and increase appetite, so I recommend limiting its use if you are sensitive to it. Processed into bulgur, it is best boiled with vegetables for about thirty minutes. (See recipe section.)

Pasta

Despite its recent vilification in the diet media, pasta is a complex carbohydrate, meaning it is slowly absorbed and provides long-lasting energy. Pasta contains significant protein—about one cup of spaghetti contains nearly as much protein as a whole egg—as well as B vitamins, iron, and fiber.

People think of pasta as fattening, but it's what is included with the pasta that causes people to put on weight. Parmesan cheese, olive oil, olives, and meatballs are the real sources of fat and calories. It's no wonder that pasta is considered a high-fat food.

The noodles themselves, even when ladled with tomato sauce (cooked without oil) and topped with vegetables, are innocent. Three and a half ounces of pasta with tomato sauce and vegetables provides about 160 calories, a little less than the same size serving of chicken and about sixty calories less than a three-and-a-half-ounce serving of sirloin steak. Unfortunately, most of us are not great at portion control, and three and a half ounces is usually just the start for any of these foods.

In order to reduce the caloric density of pasta, eat pasta with lots of fresh vegetables such as collard greens, kale, mustard greens, or broccoli. The fiber content of these vegetables will fill you up, without adding excess calories, and you'll get a healthy serving of vegetables and all of the nutrients they provide.

Fish

There's no actual need to have fish, fowl, red meat, or eggs. If you are in good condition (you exercise forty-five minutes four times a week to a sweat), you may choose to have a palm-size serving of fish (or red meat, fowl, or eggs) up to three times a week.

Fish provide a high-quality, low-fat source of protein, along with omega-3 polyunsaturated fats that lower cholesterol and protect against cancer. Always choose wild fish and avoid farm-raised varieties. I have noted below the fish that are especially rich in this important and healthy fat.

Many seafood markets, such as Whole Foods and other natural food stores, test their fish regularly for mercury or industrial pollutants. If possible, find a market that tests their fish and sells only the cleanest, freshest fish available.

Here is a list of the delicious and healthy fish and shellfish I recommend:

- Bluefish (especially rich in omega-3 fatty acids; avoid those caught in the PCB-laden Long Island Sound)
- Clams
- Cod
- Crab
- Flounder
- Grouper
- Haddock
- Halibut
- Herring (especially rich in omega-3 fatty acids)
- Lobster
- Mackerel (especially rich in omega-3 fatty acids)
- Mahi mahi
- Mussels
- Ocean perch
- Orange roughy
- Oysters
- Pollock
- Pompano
- Red snapper
- Sablefish (especially rich in omega-3 fatty acids)
- Salmon (especially rich in omega-3 fatty acids)
- Sardines (especially rich in omega-3 fatty acids)
- Scallops
- Sea bass (avoid Chilean sea bass, which is endangered)
- Shrimp
- Sole
- Squid (calamari)
- Swordfish (eat sparingly as it can be high in mercury)
- Tuna (especially rich in omega-3 fatty acids)
- Turbot
- Whitefish

Please note that I do not recommend tilapia because only farm-raised tilapia is available in the United States.

Beans and Legumes

Beans, including lentils, peas, and nuts, are all considered legumes. Beans, especially, are highly nutritious and excellent sources of B vitamins, magnesium, phosphorus, soluble fiber, carbohydrate, and protein. Beans, as I have stressed in previous chapters, are also loaded with phytochemicals, and, more specifically, phytoestrogens. Women who eat beans regularly have been found to have lower rates of breast cancer. If you are not used to eating beans, introduce them gradually to your diet.

Canned or jarred beans are fine, but choose organic varieties whenever possible.

Following is a list of the beans and bean-derived products I recommend:

- Aduki
- Black beans or black turtle beans
- Black-eyed peas
- Cannellini
- Chickpeas, also called garbanzos or ceci beans
- Fava beans
- Kidney beans
- Lentils
- Lima beans
- Miso (fermented soybean paste, rich in friendly flora that aid digestion and genistein, the isoflavone that suppresses tumors.)
- Mung beans
- Natto (whole, fermented soybeans that are used as a condiment on grains, such as brown rice.)
- Navy beans and great northern beans
- Pinto beans
- Shoyu (naturally aged and fermented soy sauce.)
- Soybeans (also called *edamame,* these are especially rich in calcium, protein, and isoflavones.)

- Soy milk (rich in isoflavones and calcium and lower in fat than whole milk, it can be used sparingly as a milk substitute. Rice milk, however, is less processed and therefore a better choice.)
- Split peas
- Tamari (a fermented soybean liquid, also rich in genistein and friendly flora, used like soy sauce.)
- Tempeh (a product made by fermenting whole soybeans, making it preferable to the highly processed tofu. It is rich in protein, calcium, isoflavones, and friendly bacteria.)
- Tofu (pressed soybeans that have had their fiber removed. Tofu is high in both protein and calcium and contains significant amounts of genistein and other phytochemicals.)

Fruit

I recommend that you eat up to two pieces of fruit per day if you are at a healthy weight and proper proportion of body fat. Serving size doesn't matter. I urge you to buy organic whenever possible and avoid fruit from Mexico and Chile because of those countries' heavy use of pesticides.

Here are my recommended fruits:

- Apples
- Apricots
- Bananas
- Berries (blackberries, blueberries, boysenberries, raspberries, strawberries, etc. These are my number-one recommended fruit, as they are low in carbohydrates and high in antioxidants.)
- Cantaloupes
- Cherries
- Cranberries
- Grapes (all colors)
- Honeydew melons
- Kiwifruits
- Mangos
- Nectarines
- Oranges

- Papayas
- Peaches
- Pears
- Plums
- Prunes
- Tangerines
- Watermelons

Dried fruit is rich in sugar and calories. Ideally, you should eat dried fruits less than once a week. If you want to eat them more often, cook them with water or fruit juice or a combination of the two.

- Dates (dried)
- Figs (dried)
- Prunes
- Raisins

Fruit spreads are permissible, as long as they contain no added sugar. Among my favorites are:

- Apple butter
- Four fruit jam
- Marmalade
- Strawberry jam

Dressings and Condiments

The following are the recommended condiments and dressings for both diets.

Oils

Remember that oil is liquid fat and drips right down to the waistline and hips. All fats contain nine calories per gram, more than twice the calories of carbohydrate or protein (each four calories per gram). Whichever oil you use, it should be organic and "cold pressed."

Organic extra-virgin olive oil is my preferred choice of fat. A tablespoon of olive oil contains 125 calories. Do not use more than one tablespoon as a dressing on salads or vegetables. If one of your health goals is to lose weight, I recommend limiting olive oil to three tablespoons per week. Otherwise, you can use up to five tablespoons per week. Olive and macadamia nut oils do not raise LDL cholesterol (the type that causes heart disease) and may slightly elevate HDL (the good cholesterol that prevents it). They are also rich in phytochemicals and may reduce the risk of some cancers: they are immune enhancing.

Other suitable oils are macadamia nut, walnut, sesame, and almond.

To keep oil quantity to a minimum, try combining smaller amounts of oil with balsamic vinegar (my favorite is Fini brand) or the juice from a freshly squeezed lemon or lime as a dressing for salads or cooked vegetables.

When using oil to sauté foods, brush the frying pan with just a thin layer of oil or add a bit of water to the pan for an olive-oil-and-water-sauté.

Coconut oil is controversial as it contains saturated fat, but it also contains medium chain triglycerides (MCTs), which are more readily metabolized.

Avoid or minimize the use of hydrogenated oils and any of the following oils, both in home cooking and in processed foods, which can be harmful because of their high saturated fat content and/or their capacity to rapidly break down and become rancid.

- Canola
- Palm kernel
- Peanut
- Soybean (the most commonly used oil in processed foods)
- Stick margarine

Vinegars

Vinegar is highly flavorful and calorie-free, making it an excellent condiment for most diets.

- Balsamic vinegar
- Japanese umeboshi vinegar (made from salted, pickled plums. Very tangy and delicious, but high in salt)
- Rice vinegar
- Wine vinegar

Other Sauces, Spices, Herbs, and Condiments

- Lemon and lemon juice
- Nasoya brand Garden Herb and/or Thousand Island Vegi-Dressings
- Pickles
- Roasted sesame seeds
- Roasted sunflower seeds
- Salsa
- Sauerkraut

Salt Substitutes

I discourage you from adding additional salt to your food at the table and recommend that you use salt only sparingly in cooking. There are a variety of healthful salt substitutes available at supermarkets and natural foods stores. Lemon juice, lime juice, and vinegar are excellent salt substitutes.

Herbs and Spices

Herbs are better for you and gentler than spices, so you should limit your intake of spices. The following is a list of recommended herbs and spices for cooking:

- Allspice. Provides a sweet and slightly salty flavor that is commonly used in soups and in fish and bison dishes.
- Anise. A licorice-flavored spice, usually used in desserts and cookies.
- Bay leaf. Provides a subtle deep, earthy flavor. Usually added to fish dishes, stews, and soups.
- Cilantro. A fresh herb common in Mexican and Asian cooking.

- Cinnamon. Used in a wide array of dishes, from oatmeal and vegetable dishes (most often squash and pumpkin) to apple pies. Fights diabetes.
- Cloves. Slightly pungent and earthy. Commonly used in desserts as well as bean and tomato dishes.
- Coriander. Sweet and spicy, it can be used in desserts, soups, salads, and stews.
- Cumin. An immune booster. Used in lentil and other bean dishes.
- Ginger (fresh, grated). An immune booster and an aid to digestion. It is pungent and sharp and used in all kinds of vegetable dishes, soups, stews, and sauces.
- Mustard. Wonderful in sauces (especially when combined with orange juice), on fish (especially salmon), and as an ingredient in sauces.
- Nutmeg. Slightly pungent and sweet. Commonly used with vegetables, especially squash.
- Oregano. Slightly pungent and aromatic. Used in fish dishes and tomato sauces.
- Paprika. Used in salads, salad dressings, soups, and in vegetable preparation.
- Parsley. Sharp tasting and rich in vitamin C, it is used in cooking vegetable and fish dishes.
- Pepper (black and white). Used to brighten dishes that are salty and savory.
- Rosemary. Aromatic and tasty. It is often used on fish, and in vegetable medleys, soups, and stews.
- Saffron. Used to prepare rice, vegetables, soups, and sauces.
- Thyme. Wonderful with fish, soups, and beans.

Nuts and Seeds

Both walnuts and almonds have been shown to lower cholesterol levels, especially LDL cholesterol, the type that causes heart disease. Walnuts contain selenium, a mineral antioxidant. Though walnuts, almonds, and sunflower seeds contain significant amounts of fat, most of it is polyunsaturated and monounsaturated. Studies have shown that people who eat walnuts and almonds tend to be more satisfied with their food and therefore tend to eat less. These people also tend to be healthier and leaner than those who do not eat nuts.

The following nuts and seeds can be eaten daily (about six whole nuts a day, not handfuls):

- Almonds
- Brazil nuts (one or two a day provides ample selenium, which has been found to be a powerful anti-cancer agent.)
- Pecans
- Sesame, squash, pumpkin, and sunflower seeds
- Walnuts

Try roasting sunflower seeds in a dry iron frying pan with raisins or other dried fruit for a delicious and satisfying snack. Add some cut-up roasted nori seaweed for added flavor and minerals.

Use the following sparingly, once a week or less:

- Cashews (high in saturated fats that raise LDL, the bad cholesterol)
- Hazelnuts
- Macadamia nuts
- Nut butters
- Pinenuts
- Pistachio nuts (avoid those treated with red dye)
- Seed butters
- Soybeans (roasted)
- Spanish peanuts

Sweeteners

Use these sparingly:

- Barley malt (especially when mixed in equal parts with a combination of brown rice syrup and water)
- Honey

- Maple syrup
- Rice syrup

Dips and Spreads

- Apple butter (try it on rice cakes!)
- Babaganoush (a Middle Eastern roasted eggplant spread.)
- Bean dips (pinto, black bean, etc.)
- Fruit spreads (choose spreads without added sugars.)
- Guacamole
- Hummus
- Salsa

Crackers

- Rice cakes

Snacks to Avoid

The following snacks are too high in calories or highly processed ingredients and should be avoided:

- Granola
- Popcorn
- Potato and other chips
- Pretzels
- Trail mix

Diet One Menu

Remember, if you are overweight, animal foods and grains should be reduced and cooked vegetables or vegetable soups increased.

I've allowed for a fairly large amount of animal foods here to help you achieve your goals without feeling deprived. Eating less meat (including fish and seafood) is always better, but it's not necessary to become a vegan to achieve good health. Those who choose to be vegan are encouraged to substitute an unprocessed whole grains combined with beans and sea vegetables wherever fish or meat are listed.

Day One

Breakfast: Scrambled Tofu (see recipe, pages 237–238); one slice
stone-   ground, organically grown whole grain spelt or whole-
wheat sourdough toast (Baldwin Hill is a fine brand); and
black, green, white, kukicha twig tea, or grain coffee (a
coffee substitute made by roasting various grains), such as
Roma, Caffix, or Pero

Lunch: Fish (three and a half ounces or about the size of your
palm) sandwich three times a week or (more preferable) a
bowl of lentil and barley soup; salad (with at least two vegetables) and dressing made from olive or macadamia nut
oil and balsamic vinegar; and tea or hot water with lemon

Dinner: Salad (with at least two vegetables) and olive or
macadamia nut oil and balsamic vinegar dressing or a
bowl of minestrone soup with lots of vegetables; brown
rice linguini and marinara sauce (with shrimp or tempeh,
if desired); broccoli rabe or steamed asparagus, sautéed in
olive oil; red or white wine; fresh or cooked (cooked is
preferred) fruit dessert; and black, green, white, or
kukicha twig tea, or grain coffee

Day Two

Breakfast: Quinoa with raisins, roasted pumpkinseeds, wheat germ
and (optional) one-fourth of a sliced apple or pear or rice
or maple syrup and black, green, white or kukicha twig
tea, or grain coffee

Lunch: Cooked vegetables with olive oil and balsamic vinegar
dressing; broiled white fish (three and a half ounces) such
as cod, scrod, or haddock (no butter used in preparation);
steamed vegetables (again, do not use butter or oil, but the
Nasoya Vegi-Dressings are a suitable and tasty alternative);
and fruit (optional)

Dinner: Miso soup (Ohsawa, South River, Miso Master, or
            Westbrae brands) with vegetables (daikon, wakame sea-
            weed, onion, or green vegetable); cooked brown rice,
            millet, or barley; steamed broccoli and kale and as many
            other vegetables as you wish; black beans with chopped
            tomato and garlic; dessert (see recipes, pages 242–244);
            and black, green, white, or kukicha twig tea, or grain
            coffee

Day Three

Breakfast: Quick-cooking amaranth, quinoa, or teff cereal (cooked in
            water or Rice Dream Vanilla Enriched Rice Milk) with
            raisins, strawberries, blueberries, or sliced banana (the
            banana only if you are physically active and not over-
            weight) and black, green, white, or kukicha twig tea, or
grain   coffee

Lunch: Salad (with at least two vegetables) with olive or
            macadamia nut oil and vinegar dressing; tempeh sandwich
            with lettuce, tomato, and mustard on organic, stone-
            ground, organically grown whole-grain sourdough bread;
            and water or tea

Dinner: Salad (with two or more vegetables) with oil and vinegar
            dressing; three-bean (organic canned is fine) salad; brown
            rice with vegetable stew; collard greens and onions sautéed
            in olive oil; water, tea, or wine; and fruit

Day Four

Breakfast: Unsweetened dry cereal, such as Kashi medley, organic
            cornflakes, or Crispy Brown Rice with rice milk or a
            cooked whole-grain cereal such as quinoa (preferred) with
            raisins or berries and black, green, white, kukicha twig tea,
            or grain coffee

Lunch: Vegetable or bean soup; bison steak or bison hamburger;
            broiled or steamed vegetables (cooked without butter);

salad (without lettuce and with at least two vegetables); fruit (optional); and tea or hot water with lemon

Dinner: Salad with two vegetables with oil and vinegar dressing (optional); grilled three-and-a-half-ounce free-range lamb chop or bison steak; steamed Chinese cabbage and button or shiitake mushrooms; and black, green, kukicha twig tea, or grain coffee

Day Five

Breakfast: Two-egg omelet (made with omega-3-rich eggs) with vegetables sautéed with as little oil as possible (use any combination of the following: onions, mushrooms, broccoli, tomato, and red or green peppers); stone-ground, organic whole-grain sourdough toast; and black, green, white, or kukicha twig tea, or grain coffee

Lunch : Brown rice, quinoa, amaranth, or millet with cooked vegetables; salad with two vegetables, with oil and vinegar dressing; water or tea; and a fortune cookie

Dinner: Beans over millet with various cooked vegetables; one or two slices organic, whole-grain sourdough bread; fruit; and black, green, white, or kukicha twig, or grain coffee

Day Six

Breakfast; Warm (not hot) Miso Soup (see recipe, page 220); warmed and moist quinoa, teff, barley, or brown rice with rice syrup or other allowed condiment (see above) if desired; cooked leafy green or vegetable medley using any of the vegetables listed above; and black, green, white, or kukicha twig tea, or grain coffee

Lunch: Minestrone soup, heavy on the cannellini beans; salad with at least two vegetables and oil and vinegar dressing fruit; and tea or hot water with lemon

Dinner: Salad with at least two vegetables and oil and vinegar dressing; kale, carrots, and onions steamed in water and olive oil; millet and chickpeas with a little cumin or curry; red wine; and dessert (see recipes, pages 242–244)

Day Seven

Breakfast: Any or all of the following fruits, cooked (preferred because cooked and warm foods quench hunger) apples, pears, prunes, strawberries, blueberries, or figs or raw (raw foods stimulate appetite) grapefruit, strawberries, blueberries, or blackberries and black, green, kukicha twig tea, or grain coffee

Lunch: Vegetable Soup (see recipe, page 217); brown rice noodles with vegetables (such as herbed baby carrots or snow peas); green leafy vegetable, such as collard greens, kale, mustard greens, or broccoli; fruit; and black, green, white, or kukicha tea, or grain coffee

Dinner: Salad with olive oil and balsamic vinegar dressing; Vegetable Soup (see recipe, page 217); seitan (if not gluten sensitive), broiled or stir-fried in three tablespoons of water and one teaspoon each of toasted sesame oil, mirin, and tamari; steamed kale and carrot medley; and black, green, white, or kukicha twig tea

Day Eight

Breakfast: Quinoa with a vegetarian milk such as almond, rice, oat, hemp, or hazelnut milk with prunes and blueberries.

Lunch: Red Lentil Soup (see recipe, page 218) flavored with aduki bean or chickpea miso; organic white or green tea

Dinner: Vegetable Soup (see recipe, page 217); salad with olive oil and balsamic vinegar dressing; Polenta (see recipe, page 225); boiled or steamed squash and carrot medley; steamed collard greens; and black, green, white, or kukicha tea, or water

Day Nine

Breakfast: Amaranth with raisins, roasted seeds, and wheat germ (sweetened with brown rice syrup, if desired)

Lunch: Miso Soup (ideally homemade—see recipe, page 220— but from a Japanese carryout restaurant is fine, too) and steamed kale with a sprinkle of roasted sunflower seeds and lots of other cooked vegetables

Dinner: Fish soup (all kinds of fish); bulgur or quinoa; baked winter squash on a bed of sauerkraut; Cucumber, Wakame, and Watercress Salad (see recipe, page 233); and two cooked vegetables with kanten (seaweed)

Day Ten

Breakfast: Scrambled Tofu (see recipe, pages 237–238): one slice stone-ground, organic, whole-grain sourdough toast; and black, green, white, or kukicha twig tea, or grain coffee

Lunch: Vegetable Soup (see recipe, page 217) or vegetable bean curd soup (you can get a double order from a Chinese carryout restaurant); Spiral Noodles (see recipe, page 227); and kale and broccoli sautéed in water and olive oil

Dinner: Millet and Cauliflower (see recipe, page 226) with canned organic (white) cannellini beans; steamed collard greens with carrots; and coffee Gelatin (see recipe, page 244)

Day Eleven

Breakfast: Quinoa, amaranth, or teff cooked in rice milk with roasted seeds and brown rice syrup and black, green, white, or kukicha twig tea, or grain coffee

Lunch;   Udon Noodles in Broth (see recipe, pages 226–227); sautéed mustard greens, onions, and carrots; and Tempeh with Sauerkraut (see recipe, page 238)

Dinner: Brown rice with Sesame Seed and Scallion Condiment
            (see recipe, page 241); broiled salmon or sardines;
            Chinese-Style Vegetables (see recipe, page 233); salad with
            your choice of dressing; and fruit

Day Twelve

Breakfast: Quick-cooking quinoa, amaranth, teff, or boxed organic
            seven-grain cereal with raisins, berries, or walnuts and
            black, green, white, or kukicha twig tea, or grain coffee

Lunch;   Vegetarian chicken or turkey salad wrap sandwich with
            lettuce, tomato, and onion; tossed salad with at least two
            vegetables; and fruit

Dinner;   Miso-vegetable soup; Soba Noodles with Sauce (see recipe,
            pages 227–228); sautéed kale and other vegetables; Black
            Beans with Onions, Carrots, and Peppers (see recipe, page
            236), and Kanten (see recipe, page 242); and fruit

Day Thirteen

Breakfast: Oatmeal, quinoa, or amaranth with raisins, toasted seeds,
            and sweetener and black, green, white, or kukicha twig
            tea, or grain coffee

Lunch: Split Pea Soup (see recipe, pages 219–220); Buckwheat
            and Bows (see recipe, page 225); and sautéed mustard
            greens

Dinner: Linguini with fish marinara; steamed broccoli rabe; salad
            with two vegetables; and fruit

Day Fourteen

Breakfast: Berries cooked in juice or rice milk and black, green,
            white, or kukicha twig tea, or grain coffee

Lunch: Salad with two vegetables and tempeh strips or beans

Dinner: Red Lentil Soup (see recipe, page 218); Polenta (see recipe, page 225); Baked Winter Squash (see recipe, page 232) drizzled with one teaspoon each of toasted sesame oil, mirin, and tamari; Arame (seaweed) with Lemon and Sesame Seeds (see recipe, page 239); steamed broccoli and cauliflower; and baked apples

Diet Two Menu

Below are two weeks' worth of menus for the Maximum Healing Diet. If you are overweight (defined as more than an inch of pinch), reduce grains and animal foods while increasing cooked vegetables and vegetable soups.

Day One

Breakfast: Quinoa, amaranth, or teff with raisins, roasted seeds, and wheat germ, sweetened with barley malt or brown rice syrup

Lunch: Sandwich on whole-grain bread filled with steamed greens (such as collards, kale, or mustard greens) and sliced tofu (seasoned with tamari, toasted sesame oil, grated ginger, and mustard or pan-roasted sesame seeds)

Dinner: Brown rice, barley, or millet; sautéed onions and cabbage; Baked Winter Squash (see recipe, page 232); Black Beans with Onions, Carrots, and Peppers (see recipe, page 236), and miso; and dried fruit cooked in apple juice

Day Two

Breakfast: Scrambled Tofu (see recipe, pages 237–238) or quinoa, amaranth, or teff cooked in sweetened and enriched rice milk and whole-grain bread with apple butter or jam

Lunch: Leftover rice; steamed watercress and carrots; and fruit

Dinner: Udon in tamari broth with shiitake, bonito flakes, and kombu; steamed kale; Tempeh with Sauerkraut (see recipe, page 238); and Coffee Gelatin (see recipe, page 244)

Day Three

Breakfast: Oat groats (cooked all night in a slow cooker)

Lunch: Chinese-Style Vegetables (see recipe, pages 233–234) served over rice or bean noodles

Dinner: Millet and Cauliflower (see recipe, page 226); steamed greens and turnips; Baked Winter Squash (see recipe, page 232); and Kanten (see recipe, page 242)

Day Four

Breakfast: Miso soup with onions, carrots, wakame, and millet

Lunch: Fried leftover millet with scallions and carrots; steamed broccoli; and any bean cooked in tamari soy sauce, ginger, and water.

Dinner: Broiled wild salmon, sole, or trout; brown rice balls (sticky brown rice mixed with chopped almonds, rolled into balls, and covered in roasted sesame seeds); salad with vinaigrette; and baked apple with cinnamon

Day Five

Breakfast: Quinoa, amaranth, or teff (cooked all night in a slow cooker)

Lunch: Hummus dip with celery sticks

Dinner: Miso soup with watercress and shiitake; brown rice, millet, and/or barley with sesame seeds; sautéed onions, carrots, and collard greens; lentils with onions, winter squash, and kombu; and fruit crisp

Day Six

Breakfast: Leftover rice (add water and cook longer for softer grain) sweetened with rice syrup or barley malt

Lunch:	Whitefish salad (whitefish mixed with vegetarian mayonnaise and a touch of tamari soy sauce and ginger) sandwich on a roll
Dinner:	Buckwheat and Bows (see recipe, page 225); cucumber and watercress salad; steamed carrots; and roasted seeds with raisins and tamari-roasted almonds (from a natural foods store)

Day Seven

Breakfast:	Whole-wheat toast with lox (go ahead, enjoy it once in a while), tomato, lettuce, and Bermuda onion
Lunch:	Vegetable Soup (see recipe, page 217) and cooked vegetables
Dinner:	Udon noodles with sautéed onions and cabbage; pinto beans; and sautéed mustard greens with sunflower seeds

Day Eight

Breakfast:	Organic cold cereal with rice milk or apple juice and gently cooked berries
Lunch:	Millet miso soup and steamed greens with daikon (a big fat white, carrot-shaped radish)
Dinner:	Broiled wild fish, bison burgers, or beans; millet, quinoa, or amaranth—or a mixture of all three; Baked Winter Squash (see recipe, page 232); sautéed bok choy; and apple kuzu (a jello substitute made with kuzu root starch)

Day Nine

Breakfast:	Last night's whole grains heated with brown rice syrup and juice or rice milk
Lunch:	Vegetable Soup (see recipe, page 217) and cooked vegetables

Dinner: Mushroom-barley soup; brown rice with gomasio (roasted and salted sesame seeds); Chinese-Style Vegetables (see recipe, page 233) with tofu; vegetable stew made with squash, carrots, onions, and burdock root; and Arame with Lemon and Sesame Seeds (see recipe, page 239)

Day Ten

Breakfast: Toast and sliced tofu with tamari and grated ginger

Lunch: A big salad with Orange-Miso Dressing (see recipe, page 242)

Dinner: Miso soup with watercress; salmon cooked with tamari, lemon juice, and toasted sesame oil; and sautéed Brussels sprouts with daikon radish and kanten

Day Eleven

Breakfast: Oatmeal with raisins, berries, and brown rice syrup

Lunch: Rice cakes with hummus and steamed vegetables or vegetable soup

Dinner: Split pea soup with barley; Baked Winter Squash (see recipe, page 232) and other vegetables; and sautéed collard greens with kale, tamari, and apple cider vinegar

Day Twelve

Breakfast: Hot cereal (seven-grain or any unprocessed, whole, slow-cooked grains in warmed rice milk or juice) and fresh fruit

Lunch: Soba or quinoa noodles with a sauce of tamari, mirin, sesame oil, brown rice vinegar, garlic, and ginger mixed with steamed broccoli and carrots with rice vinegar dressing

Dinner: Fish soup with amaranth; sautéed leeks, carrots, and rutabagas; steamed kale and onions; and coffee gelatin (see recipe, page 244)

Day Thirteen

Breakfast: Scrambled Tofu (see recipe, pages 237–238) or barley cooked in rice milk and whole-grain, organic, stone-ground bread

Lunch: Packaged ramen noodles in miso broth and salad with multiple vegetables

Dinner: Mushroom-barley soup; brown rice, barley, millet, quinoa, or amaranth with nori seaweed; Root Vegetable Stew (see recipe, pages 232–233); onion and kale sautéed in olive oil; and pinto beans with onions, carrots, and green peppers

Day Fourteen

Breakfast: Whole-grain toast with one slice of smoked salmon (lox), lettuce, tomato, and onion

Lunch: Fried rice with onions, carrots, scallions, broccoli, and nori

Dinner: Red Lentil Soup (see recipe, page 218) with beets; spiral noodles with olive oil or tomato sauce; steamed collard greens and carrots; and salad with multiple vegetables

CHAPTER ELEVEN

Week Two: Exercise for Stronger Immunity and a Longer Life

Here's a fundamental truth about health promotion that few people realize: if you are exercising, you'll find it easier to do all the other things that make your health and your life better. Exercise empowers people like no other form of activity. I like to think of exercise as the exact opposite of cigarette smoking. Just as cigarette smoking increases the likelihood of engaging in other unhealthy behaviors, exercise dramatically increases the likelihood that you will engage in all kinds of healthy activities. For example, people who exercise are much more likely to eat a healthy diet. Indeed, exercise is the single, most consistent factor in determining whether or not a person sticks to a healthy diet.

People who exercise experience less stress. They tend to be closer to their ideal weight, if not at that weight, and they are less likely to experience depression. They also maintain their youth longer and, overall, age more slowly. My experience with patients who exercise is that they tend to have greater confidence and stronger will. They are also more likely to go out and have fun. If you want to regain your health, you must commit to an exercise program.

As I discussed in Chapter Nine, it is important to have a thorough physical examination before you start any exercise program. Tell your doctor or healthcare provider that you are planning to start exercising regularly. Heed his or her advice about any limitations that you should observe regarding exercise, especially at the outset of your program. I strongly encourage you to tell your physician about the three-part exercise program that you are about to begin and ask him or her if there are any sports or activities that you should refrain from participating in. Ask specifically if you should refrain from any physical activity that requires certain types of movements, especially certain types of stretching exercises. Your health-care provider may urge you to limit your physical activity, and especially avoid competitive sports, until your fitness level improves. If that's the case, stay with the first part of this program until you are ready to move on to parts two and three.

Once you receive a clean bill of health from your physician, I urge you to adopt the program described below. A personal trainer can be a great help.

A Three-Part Program

I'm going to give you a simple program that can change your life. It consists of three primary parts, with a fourth to be added later, after you have made exercise an entrenched habit. Here is a summary of all four parts:

1. Walk daily. You can start out walking five minutes a day and add five minutes once a week building up to thirty minutes (or more). Gradually expand the distance as your fitness improves.
2. Participate in a class or game that requires skill and involves at least one other person. This activity should be done at least twice a week, preferably more. Among the best such programs are yoga, martial arts, tennis, racquetball, golf, or ballroom, tango, swing, or aerobic dancing.
3. Commit to moving your body throughout the day. Talk about it, tell others, and enlist their help. Once these three behaviors become habitual, you are ready for the fourth step.
4. Resistance or weight training. This does not mean becoming Mr. or Ms. Atlas. It means doing some simple exercises, starting with small dumbbells and ankle weights to strengthen your upper and lower body.

Allow me to lead you through all four of these transformative steps. Also, read the exercise portions at www.thepmc.org.

Step 1: Walking—The Foundation of Your Health Program

This is the first exercise that most people should start with. It requires no special skill or level of physical fitness. You can walk for as long as is comfortable, stop and rest, and then resume your walk when you are ready. In fact, you can begin with as little as five minutes a day—two-and-a-half minutes out and the same time back.

You'll need a good pair of walking shoes. Be sure they are light, well cushioned, and comfortable. Do not walk in running shoes, which are too stiff, or shoes that hurt your feet. You'll also need some loose clothing. It's a good idea to layer your clothes so that you can remove your jacket or sweatshirt, and tie it around your waist if you become too warm from the exercise.

Choose an enjoyable place to walk. You can walk around your block, at the mall, in a park, or in your local woods. It doesn't matter, as long as you feel nourished and supported by the environment. Try to avoid walking in an area where there is industrial pollution or car fumes. If you work in a city and walk at lunch, walk away from the most intense traffic. If possible, walk in a park.

Walk for, or build up to, at least thirty minutes per session, at least four to five times a week. It is fine to start with five minutes a day, five days a week and add five minutes each week.

Time is more important than distance, especially in the beginning when you are not yet physically fit.

Speed is not a factor. People who stroll still enjoy enormous health benefits from walking. Actually, I encourage people who are just starting an exercise program to walk slowly at an enjoyable pace. Do not stress yourself, either by walking too far or too fast.

Here's a self-test that you can use to see if you are pushing yourself too hard. You should be able to talk easily as you walk. If you become short of breath, slow down or stop and rest for a while.

Even though distance does not matter, I would like you to measure how far you walk. I would also encourage you to note how fast you walked. The only significance of either of these is the enjoyment of seeing your fitness improve over time. People who walk consistently for a few weeks notice that they can walk farther and faster without feeling fatigued or short of breath.

If you cannot find a thirty-minute block of time daily to walk, then walk three times for ten minutes each. The American College of Sports Medicine (ACSM) points out that even that much walking will provide health benefits and possibly life extension. Harvard University's Women's Health Study found that women who walked just one hour a week experienced half the risk of developing coronary heart disease than women who did not walk at all. That means that even a little walking each day will promote better health. Of course, if you do thirty minutes a day, you will gain even greater benefit, and you will be able to move on more quickly to step two of the program.

If you can, team up with a walking buddy so that you can keep each other motivated to take that daily walk.

Treadmills: Invest in Your Health

One of the best investments in your health you can make is to purchase a treadmill with a cushioned walking surface. I have used a wide array treadmills over the years and I prefer the Landice Treadmill, which is widely available in sporting goods shops around the country or on the Internet.

Treadmills make it possible to exercise while you watch the news or listen to music. This makes exercising a lot easier and more enjoyable. Treadmills also provide an abundance of valuable information. They tell you how far you walked, at what speed, and often how many calories you burned. Such information often motivates people to walk that extra mile, especially if they are listening to their favorite music or watching a program they enjoy. Treadmills, of course, are available at virtually every health club, along with a lot of other fun, health-promoting equipment and scenery.

Walking is the best form of exercise for people who have been sedentary and who do not currently have good physical fitness.

If you cannot afford a treadmill or a health club, then consider a stationary bicycle, which is far less expensive and is also highly aerobic. Stationary bikes can be set for greater and lesser resistance, simulating hilly terrain, or flat surfaces. Like treadmills, many stationary bikes keep track of your distance and some even report your calorie expenditure. I like the Aerobic Rider as an even better bike alternative.

My only concern about a stationary bicycle is that you can easily over-stress your heart while riding. If you are not in good cardiovascular condition, do not set the bicycle for hills. Keep the resistance light and the riding surface flat. Extra resistance can also hurt joints and tendons. Once again, see your physician for the best advice.

Walking and bicycling will train virtually all the large muscle groups. Both exercises are highly aerobic, and as long as you do not over do it, they are safe. They do not represent a complete exercise program, but either one can be the foundation of a good exercise regimen. They boost your fitness and prepare you for the next step: exercising for fun, skill, and fitness.

Step Two: For the Love of the Game

The second part of the exercise program is finding a sport, an exercise class, martial art, or other activity that requires skill and the participation of at least one other person.

Walking is a very pleasurable experience, especially when you walk in nature, but it does not provide the pleasure of participating in a game that you truly enjoy. Finding a sport, a martial art, or a yoga practice that you love, one that requires skill, fitness, flexibility, and strength, is one of life's greatest blessings. I have found that people who participate in a class or sport are much more likely to exercise for the rest of their lives. The benefits, especially when you participate with others, are innumerable.

First, you will exercise without ever thinking you're getting a workout. For example, people who love tennis find themselves getting a vigorous workout without ever thinking, "I am exercising." They aren't really exercising, they say; they're playing. It's the same for any game, martial art, or activity that you love.

I don't believe anyone will continue to exercise for a lifetime unless they find something that they truly enjoy. Exercise for the sake of exercise is too strenuous, too painful, and too tedious for most of us. And the rewards are often highly abstract, especially if you are over forty years of age and no longer buffing up your body for the opposite sex.

A game, or a martial art, or yoga, on other hand, will keep you involved because the rewards are many and instantaneous. For one, there is the opportunity to develop skills and abilities that you may not have known you have. For a tennis, racquetball, or basketball player, there is the thrill of a single good shot that you somehow performed better than you did the day or week before. For those who perform martial arts or yoga, there is the unique satisfaction that comes when a movement is performed with more grace, integrity, and power than ever before. These rewards are immediate and enormously satisfying. They keep us coming back to the game or the practice. They encourage us to improve our skills, to strengthen our bodies, and to develop our fitness all the more.

Even as you age, the game or practice keeps you young, and makes you feel even younger, because it improves your flexibility, physical strength, coordination, and stamina. And it encourages you to stay fit in order to continue to perform the game at the level you have achieved.

A game or practice that requires skill also reveals how well you are taking care of your body. You find that if you are eating well, getting a good night's sleep, and are emotionally balanced, you will perform your sport or practice better than if you are out of balance and not taking good care of yourself. Every time you engage in the practice, you get a report card on your body, mind, and emotional life. Such a sport or practice is an incentive to take better care of yourself.

Finally, these types of physical practices or sports usually involve at least one other person. This makes the practice even more pleasurable. It's a social event that will introduce you to other people or strengthen friendships that you already have.

Here are a few ideas for getting involved in a practice or sport that you can enjoy for the rest of your life:

Golf, tennis, swimming, and racquetball are all sports for a lifetime. Many health and fitness clubs offer indoor tennis and racquetball courts that allow you to play year round. There are outdoor tennis courts as well, of course. Most clubs also offer private instruction, and most recreational departments also offer adult tennis and racquetball lessons.

Recreational departments of most towns provide lessons in yoga and golf, and offer participation in adult-basketball leagues, as well. Golf is not only a great sport—if a bit frustrating at times, which is part of its mystique—but also a wonderful social event. If the golf bug bites you, you will play for the rest of your life. As long as you don't use the golf cart, the game can be a good aerobic workout, as well.

Some of the most aerobic exercises, of course, are swimming and water aerobics, both of which are offered at YMCAs, YWCAs, or Jewish Community Centers. Also, many health clubs offer pools and water aerobic classes.

Water aerobics are wonderful for people who experience joint pain, arthritis, or have old physical injuries that make exercising difficult. Water offers twelve times the resistance of air, yet it also lightens your body as you exercise. When you are chin-deep in water, you weigh one-tenth your normal body weight. When you're chest deep, you weight one-third of your body weight; when you're submerged to your waist, you weigh one-half your normal body weight. This takes most of the strain off your joints and allows you to jump up and down with far less risk of injury. Twenty to thirty minutes of water aerobics provides you with a full body workout.

Think twice before you start playing basketball, however. Basketball is intensely aerobic and sometimes extremely stressful. Only those who are in the best cardiovascular shape should take up that game. Therefore, I do not recommend basketball unless you have already done physical conditioning and are thoroughly checked out by a physician. Once you're in shape, however, basketball is one of the best games ever invented and guaranteed to keep you in shape.

Classes and dojos for karate, tae kwon do, tai chi chaun, judo, kickboxing, and other martial arts are available in virtually every city and most small towns throughout the United States. Most dojos, or places of instruction, offer both private and group lessons at extremely affordable rates. They are designed for people at all levels of athletic ability and coordination. I know several people who have never participated in sports at any time of their lives, but took up a martial art late in life and loved it. They tell me that martial arts practice is extremely empowering. It develops tremendous physical strength and confidence. It is also a way to work out issues of aggression, inner conflict, and old anger.

Yoga. Among the most widely available exercise classes today are those for yoga, aerobic dancing, and stretching classes, including Pilates. There are numerous types of yoga available for people at all levels of ability. There are classes for beginners who have never participated in any form of physical exercise. Yoga is a meditative exercise, one that gets you much more in touch with your body, mind, and spirit. Pilates is much the same and as good or better.

Dancing. There are also classes for ballroom dancing, swing, tango, African dance, and aerobic dancing. All of them are highly aerobic and require tremendous coordination. Not only will you get a wonderful workout, but also you will meet people who have similar interests to your own. It's a great way to socialize as you exercise.

Hiking clubs and nature walks. Lots of towns have organized nature walks and hiking clubs. Walking with others is a chance to make new friends and have fun while you are exercising. Consult your local recreation department for organizations that provide regular walking clubs or hiking programs.

Join the local YMCA, YWCA, or Jewish Community Center. These centers provide everything from swimming to basketball to volleyball to hiking. Call or drop by and talk to the nice people there about the programs being offered to see what works for you.

Running Is Great—But Not for Everyone

I encourage people to get involved in a sport or practice that involves other people, in part because those who exercise with others are the most likely to keep exercising for the rest of their lives.

The only exception to this rule is those who are already avid and committed runners, or those who are in the process of becoming a runner. Most people are not runners, though many people would like to be runners. A great number of people start out running but discover that it's not for them and eventually drop the whole business of running—and exercise. They feel that they failed at running and have no other recourse but to become couch potatoes.

People who give up running should realize that running is only meant for a very select group of people whose temperament and body types make running the ideal sport for them. Running is not for everyone. It's not even for most people.

On the other hand, every one of us has a sport or an activity that naturally resonates with our inner being and provides us with the rewards experienced by those who run religiously. Part of a healthy life is finding a particular sport or activity that is pure joy and fun for you, and then doing it several times a week.

A very important note: avoid competitive games if you are out of shape. If you are new to exercise, it's wise to avoid competitive games because people often forget themselves in the heat of battle. The consequence can be a fatal heart attack or an injury that sidelines you for several months.

Step Three: Move Your Body

Every day offers countless opportunities for very short bursts of activity, stretching, or movement that all combine to improve your health. Cleaning your house, your office, or your car all present opportunities for stretching and physical exercise. You can think of these everyday activities as forms of yoga.

Lunchtime offers an opportunity to take a stroll, even if it's just around the block. It moves your muscles, exercises your heart, and helps your digestion.

One of the men I greatly admired, Nathan Pritikin, used to take a short run before he ate lunch, even in places where he lectured. Before taking his place at the dining table, he would go outside and run for a hundred yards or more. He would do it with his suit on and wouldn't even bother to loosen his tie. People who wanted to talk to him would have to run beside him. Once his run was finished, he would go inside and eat his lunch. Socially, he was a little screwy, but biologically he was right: move as much as you can, not to exceed fourteen hours a day.

Life presents us with an endless array of chores that require us to be physically active. Individually, none of these movements are particularly difficult or stressful. They don't appear to add much to your fitness, but each can improve blood circulation, move the lymphatic system, massage organs, and stretch muscles. Cumulatively, these small movements can have a tremendous effect on your health, muscle tone, and weight. These little activities can contribute immeasurably to your health. The "fidget factor," just getting up and down or moving in a chair, significantly affects your metabolic rate.

Therefore, whenever possible, avoid the elevator and use the stairs. As a rule, never take an escalator, unless there are no stairs available, or you are dead tired or just plain sick. When you can, run up the stairs.

Walk at lunchtime, even if it's just for ten minutes. Bend down to pick up a piece of paper on the sidewalk. As you do, gently stretch your muscles. Every day, do four or five minutes of stretching or yoga exercises while sitting at your desk. Stand up in your office and do some gentle stretching or yoga postures. Do not tax yourself. The idea is to gently stretch your muscles, promote blood and lymph circulation, deep breathing, greater relaxation, and break out of the confined posture you may be in.

Life is constantly offering us opportunities to bend and stretch—even if it's just to pick up a dropped pen. It's constantly offering us opportunities walk a little faster, or farther, to breathe a little deeper, and to release our muscles from their habitual postures, cramps, and spasms.

These three simple steps will change your life—there is no doubt about it. They will change you in body, mind, and spirit. You will feel a thousand times better than you do right now.

After you have established a routine for walking, and you are engaged in some physical practice that you perform regularly, you will find that you are naturally more physically active in other areas of your life.

Step Four: Resistance Training

Resistance training is essential for anyone concerned about preventing bone loss or osteoporosis. Walking does not provide sufficient weight-bearing exercise for the upper body, the arms, wrists, and hands—all very important in our efforts to prevent osteoporosis. Researchers have found that people up to one hundred years of age can improve muscle fitness, bone strength, and range of motion by doing simple resistance exercises like those I describe below.

To begin a resistance training program, all you need are a pair of hand weights and a pair of ankle weights. Women should start out using three-, five-, or seven-pound hand weights, depending on starting strength and fitness. Men should start out with five-, ten-, or fifteen-pound hand weights.

Ankle weights, which come in pouches that you strap onto your ankle, come in weights ranging from one to ten pounds and can be adjusted to meet your needs.

You can perform many exercises with these simple, inexpensive weights. Do them carefully and faithfully, and you'll notice that your fitness improves quickly and steadily.

If you'd like to learn more about resistance training, the book *The Power of 10: The Once a Week Slow Motion Fitness Program* is well worth a read.

Follow these tips for starting a resistance training program:

- Be sure to start with a weight that is light enough that you can lift it easily, especially when first starting a new resistance training program.
- Breathe deeply as you do each exercise. Exhale as you lift, inhale as you lower.
- Return the weights to the floor or tabletop slowly, without losing control over the weight. If you cannot return the weight slowly and carefully, you are using a weight that's too heavy for you.
- Stop if you experience any pain, especially a stabbing pain. Do not strain yourself or overdo your workout. Use good common sense. Pushing yourself too hard will surely cause an injury. Start out slowly and do more as your fitness improves.
- Count "One, one thousand; two, one thousand . . ." up to "ten, one thousand" for each half-repetition, so that one repetition—not one set—takes twenty seconds.

The following exercises are effective for strengthening the lower and upper body:

Leg Extenders

Strap on your ankle weights and sit in a sturdy chair. Inhale and lift one leg directly out in front of you as you exhale. Hold your leg out for one second, and then lower it to its starting position. Repeat with your other leg. That's one repetition. Do five to ten reps, depending on your fitness level.

Hamstring Curls

Hold the back of a sturdy chair for support. Balance firmly on both feet. Inhale, bend your knees slightly, and raise one leg, lifting from your buttocks, exhaling as you lift. Hold for one second, and slowly release the leg to the ground. Do the same with the other leg. That's one repetition. Do five to ten reps.

Arm Curls

Sit in a sturdy chair. Take a hand weight in one hand. Rest your arm and the dumbbell on your leg or on a tabletop. Breathe in. Curl your arm with the weight toward your chest while exhaling; hold it for one second, and then slowly let it come down to your leg. (Note: senior citizens should do this exercise with a board on their lap or on a low table top to keep the weight from falling on their leg and causing an injury.) Do the same with the other arm. Do five to ten repetitions, counting twenty seconds for each rep as described above.

Wrist Curls

Hold a hand weight in one hand and rest your forearm on your leg, a board, or a tabletop. Breathe in. Curl the weight toward your body, using your wrist alone, exhaling as you lift. Do not move your arm. Just lift the weight off the tabletop, the board, or your lap using your wrist. Slowly return your wrist and weight to your lap or tabletop. Do the same with the other wrist. Do five to ten reps.

CHAPTER TWELVE

Week Three: Overcoming Stress and Developing Optimism

Most people hear the word "stress," and they automatically think of something bad and unhealthy. Actually, stress has an important purpose. Ordinary stress is meant to challenge us to bring out the best in ourselves. Chronic stress, and the unhappiness that usually accompanies it, forces us to change. Change what? You may ask. Change the underlying beliefs that keep us stuck in our stressful situations and our misery.

You could say that unhappiness is a Darwinian impulse. Unhappiness occurs when your life, livelihood, status, or identity are challenged or threatened. If the threat is chronic, or ongoing, then you feel a great need to change. Therefore, you could say that chronic stress drives us to change our lives, both inwardly and outwardly, so that we can evolve and achieve a greater degree of safety and self-expression. It forces us to become more capable of meeting our needs.

We typically think of evolution as a process by which a species survives, and that is true, but the process of individual evolution is a natural instinct to grow or evolve in order to remain successfully alive. An essential aspect of human development, or growth, is to preserve and strengthen our mental health.

Mental health is fundamental to survival. Without it, we stop perceiving reality accurately, which prevents us from successfully adapting to our environments. Failure to adapt is the primary reason a species dies out. It's also the reason many people die prematurely. They fail to adjust their belief systems, their eating patterns, their smoking habits, and other behaviors. Consequently, they end up killing themselves. Why? Because they did not perceive how important it was to change certain fundamental beliefs that made them think that they needed those hamburgers, or those cigarettes, or that job, or that relationship.

Mental health is the basis for successful adaptation. That's one reason we guard it so desperately. We need it to go on living.

Stressful situations, especially those that chronically endure, are—or should be—catalysts for changing some belief or way of behaving. In most cases, if you change fundamental beliefs, you will also change your behavior, which in turn will change your environment.

So while most people think of stress as bad or unhealthy, it really depends on how you look at it. Or, more to the point, how you react to it. If you change and adapt successfully, you can achieve a whole new level of happiness. Getting to that happiness, not dwelling on stress should be your healthful focus. The stressful situation may very well wind up being the catalyst to greater joy and satisfaction in life.

When viewed from that perspective, you may end up saying that the stress was a good thing because offered you the chance, and the impetus, to change. Many people who leave their jobs and find better ways of supporting themselves, or leave a relationship that was unhealthy, end up saying that their former problem was the best thing that ever happened to them. I hear this from patients who have overcome serious illnesses all the time. The problem becomes the catalyst to a better way of life.

Rather than look at stress as good or bad, maybe we should be asking ourselves a basic question: do we want to change in order to become happy? If the answer is yes, you're willing to change, then you have a very good chance of being happy.

Unfortunately, many people don't look at stress in this way. They believe that if they are unhappy, the world around them ought to change. The consequence of this belief is to remain stuck in pain and misery, both of which eventually lead to sickness. If you are willing to change, you can grow, evolve, and change behavior patterns so that you become much happier.

Happiness is a strange word that many people no longer believe in. I am someone who does believe in that word, but perhaps not in the way that you might think.

Happiness is just an inner condition that makes you feel safe, able to express yourself, and able to satisfy some of your most cherished needs.

Happiness and unhappiness are very temporary conditions—or at least they should be. They are nature's way of bringing us back to ourselves, of forcing us to take stock of our lives to see if anything needs changing. Happiness and unhappiness are very helpful conditions. They can be guides and stimuli for healthful growth and adaptation.

I am, by nature, a practical man. I believe that if something isn't working, you need to change it—and do so as quickly as you can. When I apply that kind of thinking to the whole subject of stress, I come to the basic belief that, in order to deal effectively with stress, you must change your behavior. That means, essentially, that the emphasis is on doing. What you do will make all the difference in the world. You can't sit around and mope about your troubles and expect your life to get better. It doesn't happen. Action is essential.

Moreover, the action has to have a purpose, or a goal. Don't meditate for the sake of meditating, or simply to say that you tried meditation. If you meditate in this way, you'll get nothing out of it. You won't be able to go deep enough to experience peace and balance.

Instead, meditate with the intention of feeling what you feel. There's incredible value in your feelings. They can guide you out of your distress. The meditations I provide below can give you greater peace and tranquility, but they can also help you discover what you are feeling.

I have the same attitude toward all healing tools: you have to use them with the clear intention of changing yourself and creating a better life. Action without purpose is pretty useless. It's just a way of fooling ourselves into thinking that we're trying to change, when we really aren't.

Basically, there are two forms of action: *yin* actions and *yang* actions. Yin actions are essentially passive, receptive, and open to new ideas. The best kinds of yin actions are listening, feeling, and learning. Yang actions are assertive, proactive, and creative. The best kinds of yang actions are remedial, meaning they address problems directly and find solutions. You need both yin and yang actions in order to succeed in your endeavor to create a better, happier life.

Let's look at the yin and yang of overcoming chronic stress.

The best place to begin to solve a problem is with the yin actions. By that, I mean listen to your inner voice; listen to others; feel your own inner impulses, desires, and frustrations; and learn what your options are. In other words, healing begins with greater self-knowledge.

The Yin Road to Freedom

The first thing to do when you are in trouble is to figure out what's going on inside. In effect, you have to explore your own feelings, beliefs, frustrations, anger, and sadness. It's essential to know what you are feeling, because those feelings are the source of your actions and your effect on others. Our inner feelings create our behavior and shape our environment. Therefore, you have to know what you are really feeling if you are going to change.

I had a patient once who was always angry. He radiated anger, and even when he didn't say a word, he intimidated people around him. Once I said to him, "Do you know that you intimidate people?"

He looked surprised. "No," he said. "Why do you say that?"

"Well, people sense that you're very angry," I said.

"Really," he said. "I don't feel angry. Are you sure people think of me as angry?"

"How do you see yourself?" I asked him.

"I see myself as a nice guy, someone who's always trying to help people."

"That's interesting," I said. "Do the people who interact with you during the day see you in that way?"

He thought for a long minute. And then he said, "Some see me that way, but I don't believe that most people see me in the way that I really am."

Now I didn't doubt for a minute that this man really was a nice guy and that he really did want to be of service to people. Like all of us, he wanted to be loved and to love. But I also perceived that he had many feelings that were unprocessed that he was unaware of. These feelings were influencing his world, nonetheless.

"Maybe you should do some self-exploration around the subject of anger," I suggested.

"How can I do that?" he asked.

"There are lots of ways," I said. "You could write in a journal, see a therapist, or talk to a minister, a priest, or a rabbi. There are lots of very good transformational programs, such as men's groups, for example, that help people get to the root of their anger and discover what it's all about. Find out why you're so angry and deal with that. Otherwise, it's going to negatively affect your relationships and limit your opportunities in life."

Write It All Out

One of the things we can all improve, I believe, is listening—listening, first to ourselves, and then listening to others. When a stressful situation arises, many people try to create safety, either by withdrawing from the situation, trying to control it, or by pleasing others. These strategies often backfire because our attempts to create safety are being motivated by fear, rather than by a true understanding of the situation and our own needs. In other words, all we understand about the situation, and ourselves, is that we are afraid of it. We don't really understand what's going on inside of us or within the situation itself.

I can't tell you how many patients come to me with some physical complaint and end up telling me that the real source of their distress is the fact that their job is in jeopardy or that they have just been laid off or fired. "Don't worry so much," I tell them. "You're going to get through this."

Of course, I offer more extensive counsel than that, but that is usually the first thing I tell them. In the vast majority of cases, I see these same people six months or a year later and they tell me that they got a better job, and they're feeling great.

"It seems like losing that job was a kind of favor," I sometimes say.

"Oh yes," the person says. "But I didn't know that at the time."

My point is that fear often keeps us from realizing how unhappy we are in certain situations and how much we need a change of circumstances. Sometimes, getting laid off or fired can be a very therapeutic and helpful thing for us.

Of course, if we don't realize how miserable we are in that job or some other circumstance that isn't working in our lives, we may never change it. This is why it's so important to allow your deeper feelings to emerge and for you to really listen to those feelings. This is the first step in dealing effectively with stress.

One of the most powerful ways of listening to yourself and discovering what you truly feel is to write in a journal. Studies have shown that people who regularly write about their feelings are able to overcome long-standing psychological distress. Writing in a diary has also been shown to increase optimism. In his book on the power of journaling, *Opening Up: The Healing Power of Expressing Emotions,* Southern Methodist University psychology professor James W. Pennebaker, PhD, describes how he discovered that deep psychological wounds could be healed by writing about them. His approach, which is based on the practice of writing about a single traumatic event over four days, has come to be known as the Pennebaker method.

Pennebaker learned about the power of journal writing when he himself became depressed and couldn't find a way out. He started writing his autobiography and, within months of starting, discovered that he was no longer depressed.

Impressed by his own dramatic turnaround, Pennebaker decided to test the power of writing on large populations of his students at SMU. He created a study in which students wrote about the most traumatic, shame-filled event in their lives for four days, for a minimum of twenty minutes per day. He had immunologists test the immune systems of his students before and after they did the program. At the same time, he created a control group of students who did not do the exercise and whose immune systems could be compared to the students who did. Pennebaker discovered that those who wrote about their most traumatic experiences had markedly stronger immune responses after they did the writing exercise.

Immunologists found that the journal writers experienced a significant increase in the number and aggressiveness of CD4 cells. Those who wrote about their traumatic events had fewer visits to the health clinic than their matched controls. The immune response was especially strong among those people who confessed feelings that they had never expressed, even to themselves. These people, whom Pennebaker termed "high disclosers," had the most remarkable improvement in CD4 response compared to all other participants.

Pennebaker maintains that more than mere catharsis is at work here. He suggests that psychological inhibition—the mechanism by which we keep things secret, even from ourselves—requires a certain degree of psychic and physical energy. As he puts it, inhibition is a demanding form of work, especially when a very painful trauma must be kept secret. Physical symptoms frequently occur from such inhibition, such as elevations in blood pressure, heart rate, breathing, skin temperature, and perspiration levels.

Pennebaker notes that these same symptoms occur when crime suspects undergo polygraph or lie detector tests. After working with polygraph experts at the Federal Bureau of Investigation, Pennebaker found that when suspects confess their crime and undergo subsequent polygraphs, they are remarkably relaxed, and all their physical symptoms related to inhibition disappear.

The release that accompanies confession occurs on psychological and physical levels. Pennebaker even found that when criminals confess during polygraph tests, they often feel bonded to their confessors; many send them Christmas cards and letters, thanking them for their help. In effect, some correction of an imbalance has occurred that releases energy and restores psychic equilibrium. With this restoration of balance come feelings of peace, tranquility, and resolution, as well as better health.

This same phenomenon occurs in people who use the Pennebaker writing method. During the first two days of writing, people experience negative emotions, such as anger, sadness, anxiety, and grief. On the third or fourth day, however, they experience feelings of relief, insight, and resolution, suggesting that they have released the inhibiting energy and integrated the traumatic events into their consciousness.

Pennebaker points out that one does not necessarily have to write about the event. Confessing it to someone else will have the same effect. This is almost certainly part of what religion, psychology, and psychiatry do.

The rules for writing such confessions are simple enough:

1. Write for twenty minutes each day, for four consecutive days.
2. Write continuously about the most upsetting experience or trauma of your entire life.
3. Don't worry about grammar, spelling, or structure of the piece.
4. Write your deepest thoughts and emotions regarding the experience. Include all the details you remember and insights into the

events. In effect, unearth the experience entirely from your psyche. Instead of repressing it, as you would normally do, pull it out from the roots.

The Pennebaker method is a very powerful tool. It can be especially effective if you have the support of a therapist with whom you can share the feelings and insights you discover by writing about your experience.

Once you have written about a single experience, move on to other events in your life that emerge spontaneously from your memory.

There are several benefits to be gained from this exercise. First, it can free you from the repressing inhibitions that keep you thinking and feeling in the same old ways. Those repressive mechanisms also keep us repeating the same behavior patterns, which is why certain kinds of experiences keep repeating themselves in our lives. The second is to gain deeper self-knowledge, which can result in greater compassion towards yourself. And finally, it boosts immune response and makes us healthier. So many illnesses have their roots in the traumas of our past.

In addition to the Pennebaker method, I highly recommend keeping an ongoing journal in which you remain in touch with your own emotional and psychological center. Life moves so fast in the modern world that we often forget our own feelings and, especially, our needs. Writing in a journal awakens us to our deeper feelings and needs that we can easily overlook and neglect. If we overlook what we want and what we need, we may end up doing things that others want and need from us instead of what we should be doing for ourselves. That, of course, can lead us into greater misery and distress.

Making discoveries about yourself frees a vast amount of energy and awakens your spirit in ways that no other activity or behavior can. Suddenly, you see yourself in an entirely new light. A feeling of vitality and excitement arises within you. There is hope, optimism, and a fresh wind in your sails. It's as if a door opens, and you are ready to walk through it. New opportunities start to appear, in part because you are now much clearer about who you are and what you want from your life. That alone creates a rising energy and enthusiasm for life. Writing in a journal is one of the most effective ways of making such discoveries. (For more information, visit the Psychological/Spiritual Health section of our website at www.thepmc.org.)

Meditation: The Peace Derived from Within

Another yin tool for self-exploration and healing is meditation. Meditation has a powerful effect on stress levels and immune responses.

Keep in mind that stress occurs only because we have some negative belief that keeps us unstable both in the present and for the future. That negative belief turns an "ordinary situation" into a "problem." One of the primary differences between an ordinary situation and a problem is fear—fear of how the situation will turn out.

Meditation relieves us of that fear by bringing us back to the present. Right now, you're probably fine. In fact, in the present, we're almost always fine. The only exception, of course, is if we are in immediate danger, like crossing the street as an oncoming truck hurtles toward us. Suddenly, our heart rate, respiration, and muscle activity increase. We are capable of rapid movement, which we use to run across the street to get to safety. Once we are safe, we quickly stop worrying about the truck and our near-death experience. Instead, we start thinking about our problems again, which worries us and causes us distress. Dread is well treated by healthy distraction.

One of the ways we can do that is by coming back to our breath and awakening to the present. Following is a meditative technique for doing that.

Watch Your Breath

Sit on a comfortable chair in a peaceful place within your home or office. Take off your shoes. Close your eyes, exhale a long breath, and let your shoulders drop. With each exhalation, allow the tension that is in your body to be expelled. Feel the tension go out of your body with each out-breath. Take your breath deep into your abdomen so that your stomach rises and falls with each inhalation and exhalation. Once you have reached a relaxed state, let your breath resume a normal, effortless pace. Don't force your breath, but rather allow it to assume a natural rhythm of expansion and contraction. Concentrate on each inhalation and exhalation. Listen to your breath.

As thoughts rise and fall from your mind, just witness them and then let them drift away. Meanwhile, keep your focus on your breath and your body. If your mind pulls you into some drama or inner dialogue, notice it and come back to your breath. Come back to your body. Come back to the now. You are safe. All is well. Let that safety cause your lower back and pelvis to relax. Allow any positive feelings that may arise out of that awareness of safety in the here and now to emerge. Experience your body relaxing and sinking ever more deeply into that feeling of comfort, and the positive emotions that naturally emerge from your sense of safety. If you are reading this with feeling, you'll start to notice it right here.

Once you have reached this deep state of relaxation, allow any emotions to emerge. Do not judge or repress those emotions. Rather, hold them, as it were, with your awareness, as if you were holding a child. Let the emotion inform you of how you feel. Let yourself become aware of any insight that may want to emerge. Hold that state of awareness for as long as you can, and then gradually come back to normal consciousness when you are ready.

Do this exercise for fifteen to twenty minutes every morning and every night.

Whenever you are under stress at work, pause, drop your shoulders, exhale, and come into the present. Listen to your breath sounds. Come into the present. That's where your power is. You can control your emotions and concentrate far better if you stop thinking about the future and start living in the present. The present is where safety lies.

As you become more practiced in this meditative technique, you will find that you can use it at virtually any moment of the day. You will also find those feelings of peace and tranquility that are always inside of you, and always available to you, through this meditation.

Progressive Relaxation Technique

Herbert Benson, MD, the famed mind-body researcher from Harvard University, discovered what he called "the relaxation response," in which respiration, heart rate, and hormone levels all came into balance as a result of meditative or relaxation exercises. Other common effects associated with the relaxation response are deep feelings of peace, safety, and hope, increases in brain levels of endorphins, and a greater sense of one's connection to life. Meditation and the relaxation response are both associated with significant improvements in immune function. The following meditative technique is a powerful healing tool.

This is progressive relaxation exercise can elicit the relaxation response as documented by Dr. Benson. Sit in a comfortable chair in a peaceful place in your home. Take off your shoes. Close your eyes, exhale, and drop your shoulders. Allow the tension in your body to be released with each exhalation. Feel the tension drain from your body. Breathe deeply into your abdomen, allowing your abdomen to swell and then comfortably relax. Turn your attention to your face and allow all the tension to drain from your facial muscles. Feel your face assume a much more peaceful and content countenance. Become aware of your neck and any tension you may be holding there. Exhale and let the tension go. Gently turn your head slightly to the left and then to the right, releasing the tension from your neck even more. Shift your attention down to your shoulders. Feel the condition of the muscles and tendons in your shoulders. Breathe into your shoulders; see them rise as your chest swells and then let them fall as you exhale. Let any tension that you feel in your shoulders go as you breathe out. Let your shoulders drop, releasing any tension or resistance from them. Move your awareness down to your biceps and triceps, the muscles in your upper arms. Let them drop, so that the muscles deeply relax. Keep breathing. Move on to your forearms. Notice how they feel. Breathe in and then exhale. Picture all the tension that may be in your arms, wrists, hands, and fingers draining out of your body through your fingertips.

Bring your awareness back to your chest. Breathe in and feel your chest rise and fall. Feel the muscles and organs in your chest relax. Visualize your heart coming into a state of peace and tranquility. Picture your lungs filling with life-giving oxygen. Visualize the carbon dioxide being expelled with every exhalation. As the carbon dioxide leaves your body, feel your body release any tension or pain that may be in your chest. Continue to breathe. Visualize the inhalation of oxygen as a light-filled, life-giving energy. Imagine it swirling through your chest, abdomen, and lower organs.

With every exhalation, release any tension, pain, or discomfort that may be present in your abdominal cavity. Don't worry if the tension or pain is not fully released. Just continue to witness it without distress. Let your body take in the oxygen and release the carbon dioxide. Let the wisdom of your body heal itself at its own pace.

See the life-giving energy that you inhale channeling down through your digestive organs, giving your small and large intestines all the vitality and power they need to function optimally. Note any stirrings that may be occurring in your digestive system.

Become aware of your pelvis and the organs within it. Breathe deeply into your pelvis. Exhale all the tension, discomfort, or pain that may be held there. Feel the small of your back relax. Continue to breathe. Feel your hips relax. Feel your buttocks relax. Feel your upper thighs relax. Breathe the life-giving energy into your pelvis, and visualize your entire pelvic region swelling with this energy. Exhale all the tension, and feel your muscles and organs relax even more deeply. Visualize the organs of your pelvis being healed by the light-filled, life-giving energy that you take in with every breath.

Become aware of your thighs and calves. Feel any tension in your legs. Breathe deeply into your legs, and let the energy that is within each breath travel down into your legs and feet. With your mind's eye, see your legs fill with light, energy, and vitality. Watch that light and energy enter your feet and flow into your toes. Feel your legs and feet relax. Feel yourself anchored to the earth by the energy that you take in with each breath.

Become aware of your complete state of relaxation. Continue to breathe. Observe and let go of any thoughts that may enter your mind. Watch them as they fade from view. Bring your awareness back to your breath. Feel the peace that now engulfs your body and mind.

You are now in a deep state of relaxation. Become aware of the vitality and energy that fills your being. You can direct that energy to any place within your body to support your healing. Send that energy to the places that need support. Continue to breathe. Remain in this state for as long as you like.

When you are ready, slowly and peacefully bring your awareness back to the room and resume your normal activities. It helps to reread this several times.

Ten or twenty minutes of this exercise daily will create a deep state of relaxation. It will boost your immune system and promote healing. It will make you feel more grounded, centered, confident, and powerful.

In addition to meditation and relaxation techniques, of course, is prayer. Those who feel moved to pray find this one of the most comforting and faith-inducing practices of all. It may be best to pray after you have meditated or done your relaxation routine. This is the time when you are most relaxed, clearest of mind, and most capable of articulating your needs and wants.

Regular (Twice a Month) Massage

In addition to listening to ourselves, it's important to receive the support and healing assistance of others. During times of stress, it's very easy to forget yourself and your own needs. Safety and security very often become the primary objectives. We forget that there's a lot more to us than our fears. And those fears are constantly creating muscle tension, which in turn reduces blood flow, alters the balance of hormones in our bodies, and blocks lymph from flowing optimally.

Stress is held in the tissues. That means that you've got to work with those tissues to relieve the body of the accumulating effects of stress. One of the best ways to do that is through regular massage.

There are many different forms of therapeutic massage. Among the best are shiatsu and acupressure. They are essentially the same practice, except that they originate from different countries. Shiatsu is the Japanese version of the Chinese acupressure. Both are based on the theory that there are hundreds of points—known as acupuncture points—on the body that act as generators of electrical current. That current runs along discreet pathways, known as meridians.

Each meridian serves as a kind of electrical pathway for a specific organ or system. There are fourteen pathways, or meridians, ten of which correspond to organs. These include meridians for the liver, gall bladder, heart, small intestine, spleen, stomach, large intestine, lungs, kidney, and bladder. There are four more meridians that serve as unifying pathways that integrate and balance energy among various organs and systems. These are the conception vessel, which runs down the center of the body;

the governing vessel, which runs up the back; the triple heater or triple warmer meridian, which also runs down the shoulders and along the arms; and the heart governor, which runs down the inside of the arms.

According to acupressure theory, illness occurs when a meridian is blocked or stagnant, therefore depriving individual organs and tissues of an adequate flow of energy, also known as life force or *Qi* (pronounced "chee"). Healing takes place when the energy is unblocked and flows abundantly to the affected organs or systems.

There are many other forms of therapeutic massage, among them Jin Shin Jyutsu, a Japanese healing art that also uses acupuncture points, known as safety energy locks, to stimulate the flow of energy along pathways, known as flows. Swedish, therapeutic, deep tissue and healing touch are all forms of massage that can promote improved blood and lymph circulation, unblock tension and stagnation, and cause deep relaxation to the body. These are indeed healing arts.

Massage is a way of caring for the body. It is highly therapeutic and deeply nourishing. Many doctors, myself included, refer patients to good massage therapists and alternative healers. Ask your doctor for a referral. You might also check with your health club as many gyms employ their own massage therapists or have a relationship with a separate massage practice to which they regularly refer clients. Alternative healing practices and massage therapists also often place ads in local weekly or monthly newspapers, or on the bulletin boards of local natural foods stores.

I recommend getting a massage at least twice a month, if possible. There are many forms of self-massage, as well. But anyone who lives with another person can give and receive a twenty- to thirty-minute massage at least once a week. It's free, and it's a wonderful way of expressing love. You'll both be healthier for it, as well.

One of the most important things to do during times of stress is to create a support network that includes various types of healers and counselors—physical, emotional, and spiritual. Physician healers, psychotherapists, priests, ministers, and rabbis are available for one-on-one counseling. Your doctor or healthcare provider can offer sound medical advice, dietary or nutritional counselors can advise you on making changes to your diet, and a trained holistic healer can guide you in incorporating alternative healing tools into your life. You will feel supported in ways you never dreamed possible.

These yin practices are among the most powerful tools for opening yourself up and receiving the guidance and support that others have to offer. Once you have done that, it's time to take the yang path, the path of proactive action.

Two Yangs Make a Right

The first two yang activities that everyone should take up if they want to deal effectively with stress are a healthy diet and regular exercise. These two practices alone are going to reduce, and darn near eliminate, much of the stress in your life.

The reason, very simply, is that both of these practices make you realize how much power you have to transform your life. A diet that is based on unprocessed whole foods, without the excess consumption of stimulants, such as coffee, and depressants, especially alcohol, is going to make you healthier and more balanced. Your body will no longer be dealing with the extreme highs and lows that naturally occur on the standard American diet, which is so rich in fat, processed foods, artificial ingredients, sugar, caffeine, and alcohol.

A healthy diet will make you feel more energetic, more physically alive, and clearer of mind. It will help you lose weight. You will look and feel younger, which will lead you to feel better about yourself in virtually every respect.

A regular exercise program, of the type just described, can boost your mood, give you far more energy, and greatly increase your physical power. It can dramatically increase your confidence, your will, and your personal sense of power. These two practices, diet and exercise, can transform your life all by themselves.

Change your way of eating and start exercising every day, and pretty soon you will realize that you have the power to create a better life. Then you will be ready for the next step in your healing: confronting the actual problem you are dealing with.

There is no other way around it, actually. No matter whether it's your job, your primary relationship, your financial life, or your desire to achieve certain goals and ambitions, the source of your stress must be confronted if you are to be truly healthy. If you have followed the program I've outlined above, you already have all the tools you need to confront that problem.

You have written in a journal, meditated, prayed, consulted healers, and worked with your issues. You are eating well and exercising. You're more fit, and you are experiencing much more clarity in your thinking. You are emotionally more centered and balanced. All that's left to do is to tackle your life's problems courageously.

And One More Thing ...

Put a smile on your face; laugh a lot. Watch funny movies or videos online, read funny books, listen to funny shows on the radio. That little smile and your hearty laugh will change your feelings about life and yourself. But don't forget: you're being the bravest, most enlightened version of who you are. Be proud of yourself. Sing a happy song like "I'm Looking Over a Four-Leaf Clover" (believe it or not, this happens to be the only song I know!). You're already a success.

CHAPTER THIRTEEN

Week Four: Creating Balance in Your Life

In order to establish balance in your life, you must answer the question, "Where do imbalances in my life come from?"

The most common source, of course, is fear, which is usually referred to as stress. The more fear we experience, the more imbalanced our lives become. While stress is the primary source of imbalance for most people today, there are many other sources. Sickness and disability, either our own or that of a loved one; financial problems; loneliness; inability to determine what we want to do with our lives; and drug and alcohol abuse all contribute to stress. Most of these problems trigger their own unique fears.

Many things change in our lives when fear becomes chronic. Many people spend a lot of time focusing on the problem, without doing much about it. They just think about it all the time.

Thinking without action only serves to make the problem bigger and more debilitating. It's like rubbing a wound without ever giving it the time and right conditions to heal. Other people attempt to escape the problem, often by consuming excessive amounts of sugar, watching television for long hours, or by turning to drugs and alcohol. None of these behaviors address the problem, which is why it typically gets worse. Even those who actually face a problem, but spend most of their waking hours dealing with it, are engaging in an extreme reaction to stress. In fact, all of these behaviors can be regarded as extreme, and all of them usually lead to illness, which is why creating balance is so important for all of us.

You create balance by thinking and behaving in ways that are different from those behaviors that got you into the jam in the first place. It's that simple.

Acting differently can—and must—be simple. Don't indulge in too much thinking about the problem without acting. It's very possible to overanalyze the issues and remain stuck in those issues. Overanalyzing yourself can be a disguise for your fear of taking risks and behaving in new ways. So commit yourself to restoring balance, and solving your problem, by taking different types of actions.

Here are some very simple things you can do to restore balance, and in the process, create a whole new life for yourself.

Get Help

No one overcomes any serious issue alone. Very often, we are afraid to seek help. Deal with the fear, or don't, but get help anyway. Seek out two forms of help. First, find a healer who can work with your physical, emotional, and psychological condition and help guide you toward a new way of being. Second, seek out expert advice in the specific area of your problem.

Many highly trained experts, including people who have retired from their field, provide free counseling for specific issues. There are also support groups that provide specific forms of support for all kinds of challenges. Among the best ways to find the right experts and support groups is to ask the advice of a priest, minister, or rabbi; your doctor; your lawyer; or your friends. Another great source is your local newspaper.

It's my belief that virtually every problem has a solution. Our responsibility is to sincerely and actively search for the solution. As we do, we are inevitably introduced to people who can guide us to the right sources of information, or to people who can assist us. Searching is the key to finding the answers.

Grow by Doing the Thing You Always Wanted to Do

There are things that you have always wanted to do, but were afraid to take up. There are places in the world that you have always wanted to visit. Perhaps you wanted to learn a foreign language, write a book, take up a sport or a hobby, learn to play an instrument, or study a subject that has always fascinated you.

Start doing what you have always yearned to do, even if you are doing it only as a hobby for a few hours per week. I know the CEO of a company, extremely active in the business world, who only a few years ago decided to learn to play the piano. He is sixty-three years old. Recently, he told me that he has not had so much fun, nor felt so rewarded and inspired by anything he has done in the last thirty years.

In fact, he has a talent for the instrument. But because he told himself for all of his adult life that he couldn't play, didn't have the time, or that taking up the piano this late in life would be a waste of time, he postponed an activity that today gives him enormous pleasure and satisfaction. Do what holds your interest.

I know another man who recently began studying French. He always wanted to learn how to speak French, but he was afraid to take up the language because he did miserably at language in high school and was later told that you can't learn a language as an adult. Of course, that's nonsense; you can learn anything you want to learn. Today he speaks French very well, and that makes him feel great about himself.

Do just one thing that you have always wanted to do, and new worlds— both inside and outside—will open up to you.

Create Internal Balance with Dietary Change

An essential step in restoring balance is to strengthen your own sense of center and equilibrium. Certain foods and drinks make that impossible. Therefore, I recommend the following dietary changes in order to restore your sense of self, personal power, and feelings of control:

1. Stop drinking coffee. Coffee not only contains significant amounts of caffeine (about a hundred and fifty to two hundred milligrams per cup, depending on how it's brewed), but also contains oils that cause tremendous muscle tension and stomach acidity. The physical side effects of drinking coffee make it very difficult, if not impossible, to feel balanced and centered in your own power. People who drink multiple cups of coffee every day tend to experience tremendous levels of anxiety and nervous and muscle tension.

Instead of coffee, drink a high-quality black, green, or white tea in the morning. These contain only small amounts of caffeine, along with lots of health-promoting antioxidants and phytochemicals. For an easy transition, start out using two bags of English Breakfast tea in one cup of hot water to replace one cup of coffee. Tea does not contain the anxiety and tension producing chemicals that coffee does. It will give you a boost, while at the same time helping you feel relaxed and balanced.

2. Eliminate or reduce alcohol consumption. Alcohol is a depressant. It clouds judgment and makes people feel physically weaker, even after the buzz wears off. It is also a powerful source of oxidants, which means it promotes much more rapid aging and the onset of disease. As mentioned previously, alcohol, in any dose, is toxic to heart muscle, brain tissue, and bone marrow. I recommend no more than one drink per day for women and two per day for men. Ideally, no one should drink more than four glasses of wine (or equivalent) per week.

3. Eliminate added sugar and processed foods from your diet. Eat whole grains and lots of cooked vegetables every day. Let beans be your protein and cooked fruit your treat.

Strengthen Your Will with Exercise

Adopt the exercise program described in Chapter Twelve. Find time for a walk every day. Pick up the old tennis racquet or golf clubs, or attend a yoga, martial arts, or dance class, and start playing again. Leap at opportunities during the day to exercise your body. All of these activities will strengthen your will and your personal power to transform your life. In a very real sense, they will give you back your life.

Take the Following Ten Steps to Nourish Yourself

Very often, people think that they have to make some earth-shaking change in their lives in order to restore harmony and happiness. They tell themselves, "Get out of your job," or "Break up your marriage," or "Move to another city." Such decisions are so far-fetched that they often prevent the person from making the small moves that really could make a huge difference in their lives.

Start with "baby steps." I believe in the small things, myself. I believe that if you change your diet, start exercising, and do the small things I have listed below, you will transform your life. And then very big things can happen for you. But the big things cannot happen if you don't do the little things first, because if you don't change yourself, the big life changes that you might make—quitting your job or breaking up—will only bring about another lousy job or another failed relationship. Change yourself first and see how much your external life changes.

Start to change yourself by eating more healthfully and exercising daily. At the same time, give yourself what you need to be happy.

Here are ten activities that you can use to change your life, without having to hit it with a wrecking ball:

1. Practice doing nothing. Schedule an hour or two a week to do nothing. And do it in a really relaxing place, away from people. Stroke your cat; sit in the afternoon sun; let your inner life bubble up into your consciousness and inspire you with new ideas, new dreams, and new forms of enlightenment. Doing nothing opens you up to feelings and inspirations that can only be experienced in the quiet, gentle moments of your life. These moments are like a spring of healing waters that flows within you.

2. Watch no television for a week or longer. Liberate yourself from the boob tube. Not only will it free up time, it will give you back your sense of self. Get your news from the newspaper. Reading is a wonderful and relaxing pastime. And it's much healthier than that tension-producing cathode-ray tube.

3. Schedule romantic time with your partner and play time with your children. Regularly schedule a breakfast, intimate lunch, or romantic dinner with your spouse or lover. Commit to spending more time together and enjoying your lives. Couple these dates with activities you both enjoy. Schedule a lunch or time with your children away from your home. Schedule activities that you know your child especially wants to do.

4. Get more sleep. Many of us are sleep-deprived. The body heals itself during sleep. Many people find that when they get adequate sleep, they wake with creative solutions to pressing problems. In any case, more sleep usually means better health, greater energy, and much more clarity of mind. Make rest a priority. During the week that you abstain from watching television, go to bed an hour or two earlier to catch up on sleep. An hour of sleep before midnight is worth two hours of sleep after midnight.

5. Reach out and make a friend. Call that person with whom you've wanted to develop a friendship and invite him or her to play tennis, watch a film, have a cup of tea, or otherwise spend some social time. Expand your social life by developing deeper and richer friendships.

6. Express your gratitude. Tell people how much you appreciate them, especially your spouse or lover and your children. Point out how what you appreciate about each of them and let them know how much you admire their talents. Write letters to people with whom you haven't spoken in years. Tell them what a difference they made in your life. All it takes is a card or note, expressing a small sentiment of appreciation. Support and enrich the lives of those around you, and your world will turn into a beautiful and loving garden. We are, after all, here to serve.

7. Express yourself artistically. Turn your life or your dream into a beautiful picture. With colored pencils, pens, or paints, create a picture of your inner world or how you want your life to develop. What does the next step in your life look like? Do you see yourself breaking free, becoming more relaxed, or achieving some great dream? Draw an image that expresses that feeling or shows what your life would look like if you had already accomplished this goal. Give yourself a clear picture of the future and that future will start to unfold before you. This is a surprisingly therapeutic exercise, one that will give you much more peace, tranquility, and optimism.

8. Reward yourself with tenderness and health. Give yourself a special gift that's meant to pamper you: a facial, a manicure, a

pedicure, time in a hot tub, an acupuncture treatment, an energy healing session, a night of dancing, tickets to a special event, or a weekend in the country. Think about how you would like to reward yourself for all the hard work and good that you are doing for yourself and in the world.

9. Get a lifelong friend: adopt a dog or cat from a local animal shelter. Numerous studies have shown that pets reduce blood pressure, boost immunity, and promote healing. Pets offer unconditional love and comfort, and they may even help you live longer. Certainly, you will derive much happiness from having a pet in your life.

10. Develop your own spiritual practice.

These are the little things that change your life by restoring balance to it. Balance makes it possible for you to enjoy your life and restore your connection with yourself. In other words, it is the basis of a fulfilled and happy life.

Conclusion

In this book, I have tried to show how you can unlock your body's powerful immune and cancer-fighting defenses. You do not have to be a victim of disease.

Not only can you prevent serious illness, but you also have the power to overcome it. Much depends on your behavior and your willingness to act in ways that support your immune system and your overall health.

In this book, I have provided the tools to do exactly that. The dietary, lifestyle, and psychological approaches described here can be the basis for a restoration of your good health. Indeed, it is my sincere hope that they become the basis for a new way of living. Enjoy The Preventive Medicine Center website, www.thepmc.org.

CHAPTER FOURTEEN

Recipes for Maximum Healing

Included here are more than fifty delicious recipes, all of which can boost your immune and cancer-fighting systems. These are delicious foods that can make you healthier and happier—and may even extend your life. Cook with intention and enjoy.

More recipes can be found on our website at www.thepmc.org.

Soups

Vegetable Soup

1 piece kombu, soaked and cut into small strips

1½ cups diced carrots

½ cup diced daikon radish

1 pinch salt

6 cups water

1½ cups thinly sliced leeks

2 tablespoons soy sauce or miso

Fresh parsley for garnish

Place kombu, carrots, and daikon in a saucepan. Add salt and water, and bring to a boil over high heat. Reduce heat to medium-low and simmer for 15 minutes. Add leeks and raise heat if necessary to return to a boil. Reduce heat to medium-low and simmer for 8 minutes. Add soy sauce or miso (if using miso, stir it first with a small amount of the hot soup so that it dissolves) and simmer (do not boil) for 5 minutes more. Serve immediately, garnished with fresh parsley.

Serves 4.

Red Lentil Soup

2 teaspoons organic extra virgin olive or macadamia nut oil

1 large onion, sliced

1 cup red lentils, washed and drained

6 cups water

1 bay leaf

2 medium carrots, sliced in half-inch rounds

2 beets, sliced in half-inch crescents

¼ cup dark miso

2 tablespoons toasted sesame oil

Croutons for garnish

In a soup pot, heat the oil over medium heat. Add onion and sauté, stirring regularly, for five minutes. Add lentils, water, bay leaf, and bring to a boil. Simmer for 40 minutes. Add the carrots and beets and continue simmering for another 20 minutes or so, until the vegetables are soft. Remove and discard bay leaf. Transfer soup to a blender or food processor (in batches, if necessary), puree, and return to soup pot. In a small bowl, combine miso with a little bit of the hot soup and stir to dissolve. Add miso mixture to the soup along with the sesame oil. Garnish with croutons and serve.

Serves 3 to 4.

Red Lentil and Corn Chowder

2 teaspoons sesame, organic extra virgin olive, or macadamia nut oil

1 medium onion, diced

1 clove garlic, minced

3 carrots, diced

Kernels cut from 2 ears of corn

½ teaspoon sea salt

1 teaspoon each fresh thyme, basil, sage, and rosemary (or substitute
    ½ teaspoon dried of each)

6 cups vegetable stock or water

½ teaspoon black pepper (optional)

1 cup red lentils

¼ cup shoyu or soy sauce

Thinly sliced scallions or chopped parsley for garnish

Heat oil in a large pot over medium-high heat and sauté onions, garlic, carrots, and corn with salt until onions are translucent, about 3 to 4 minutes. Add herbs, water or stock, pepper (if using), and lentils. Bring to a boil. Reduce heat to medium-low and simmer for about 30 minutes, until lentils are soft. Add shoyu and simmer for another 15 minutes. Garnish with scallions or parsley and serve.

Serves 4.

New England Fish Chowder

1 tablespoon sesame or organic extra virgin olive oil

1 medium onion, minced

1 carrot, minced

1 large stalk celery, minced

2 cups cooked rice (or substitute barley, millet, or quinoa)

6 cups water

Sea salt or shoyu soy sauce to taste

12 ounces white fish, cut into 1-inch pieces

1 teaspoon ginger juice

Chopped parsley for garnish

In a skillet over medium-high heat, heat oil with a small amount of water. Add onions, carrots, and celery and sauté for 5 minutes. Add rice, water, and either sea salt or shoyu. Simmer for 30 minutes. Add fish, cover, and let cook for another 10 to 15 minutes. Stir in ginger juice, garnish with parsley, and serve.

Serves 4.

Split Pea Soup

1 cup split peas, washed and drained

6 cups water

1 stick wakame

1 onion, diced
1 carrot, diced
1 celery stalk, diced
Tamari or soy sauce to taste

Place peas, water, and wakame in a soup pot and bring to a boil over medium-high heat. Reduce heat to medium-low and simmer for about 1 hour, or until the peas are soft. Add onions, carrots, and celery and cook for 20 minutes more. Add tamari or soy sauce to taste and serve.

Serves 3.

Miso Soup

Be careful to keep this soup at a simmer (not a boil) once the miso has been added. Feel free to substitute different vegetables and, if you wish, add millet at the beginning of cooking and cook for 30 minutes before adding the vegetables.

4–6 cups water
¼ cup dried wakame, washed, soaked for 3–5 minutes until soft, and cut into bite-sized pieces
1 medium carrot, cut into matchstick-sized pieces
1 cup thinly sliced white cabbage
½ cup thinly sliced onions
1–3 tablespoons barley, brown rice, or aduki bean miso*
Thinly sliced scallions for garnish

Bring water and wakame to a boil in a soup pot, cover, and simmer over medium-low heat for 8 to 10 minutes. Add carrots, cabbage, and onions to the pot, raise heat to medium-high, and return to a boil. Reduce heat to medium-low and simmer for 8 minutes. In a small bowl, combine the miso with a small amount of the soup and stir to dissolve. Stir miso mixture into soup and simmer over low heat for 3 minutes more. Garnish with scallions and serve.

* I recommend miso pastes made by Ohsawa, South River, Westbrae, and Miso Master.

Serves 6.

Whole Grains

Brown Rice or Barley

Soaking the grain overnight reduces the cooking time by half.

1 cup brown rice or barley

2 cups water

2 pinches sea salt (such as Celtic Sea Salt or Sal del Mar sea salt)

Wash rice or barley several times, until water runs clear. Drain.

Place rice or barley, water, and salt in a medium saucepan, cover, and bring to a rolling boil over high heat. Reduce heat to low and simmer for 45 to 60 minutes until grains are tender.

Serves 2–3.

Brown Rice Balls

Salt to taste

2 cups cooked brown rice (see above)

4 umeboshi plums, sardines, tamari, or soy sauce to taste

Drape plastic wrap in a small bowl. Add a bit of water to the bowl to wet the plastic wrap then sprinkle salt over the water. Scoop ¼ of the cooked rice onto the wet plastic wrap in the bowl, pressing it to conform to the shape of the bowl. Use a finger to create a tunnel in the rice, then fill the tunnel with an umeboshi plum, a sardine, or a bit of tamari or soy sauce. Twist the Saran wrap around the rice firmly, slowly squeezing out all of the air, to form a ball. Peel off plastic wrap. Repeat with the remaining rice and serve immediately.

Makes 4 rice balls.

Barley with Mixed Vegetables

1 cup barley, washed and soaked for 6–8 hours

1½ cups water

Pinch sea salt

½ cup fresh corn kernels

½ cup shelled fresh green peas
½ cup diced carrots
¼ cup roasted sunflower seeds
Thinly sliced scallions for garnish

Place barley and water in a pot. Add sea salt, cover, and place over high heat. Bring to a boil and reduce heat to medium-low. Cook for about 50 minutes, or until grains are tender.

While the barley is cooking, bring a pot with 3 to 4 inches of water to a boil. Add corn and cook for 1½ to 2 minutes, then remove corn with a slotted spoon and set aside to cool. Repeat this process with the peas (cooking them for 1½ to 2 minutes), and finally the carrots (cook for 1 minute).

When barley is cooked, remove from heat and let sit, uncovered, for about 5 minutes, then transfer to a serving bowl. Add the cooked vegetables and sunflower seeds and stir to mix. Serve garnished with scallions.

Serves 4.

Confetti Brown Rice Salad

1 cup brown rice
2 cups water
Pinch sea salt
1 tablespoon umeboshi vinegar
2 tablespoons brown rice vinegar
1 tablespoon apple juice
2 tablespoons sesame oil
½ cup minced scallions or red onion
½ cup fresh corn kernels, blanched
½ cup sliced snow peas, blanched
½ cup onion, diced and marinated in umeboshi vinegar for 1 hour
½ cup diced carrots, blanched

Place rice in pot, add water and salt and bring to a boil. Reduce heat to low and simmer for 60 minutes. When rice is finished cooking, immediately remove it from the pot and fluff with chopsticks or a fork. Set aside to cool.

While rice is cooking, make the dressing. In a small saucepan, combine vinegars, apple juice, sesame oil, and scallions or onion and heat for 2 minutes over medium heat. Set aside to cool.

In a large serving bowl, combine cooled cooked rice, blanched vegetables, and dressing. Toss to mix well and serve.

Serves 4–6.

Millet "Potato Salad"

3¾ cups water

1 cup millet, washed and drained

1 onion, diced

1 large dill pickle, diced

1 teaspoon fresh or dried dill

½ teaspoon celery seed

4 tablespoons Follow Your Heart Vegenaise (mayonnaise substitute)

In a saucepan over high heat, bring water to a boil and add millet. Reduce heat to low, cover, and simmer for 40 minutes.

While millet cooks, mix onion, pickle, dill, celery seed, and Vegenaise in a large mixing bowl and set aside.

When millet is cooked, spread it in a rectangular baking dish and refrigerate, uncovered, until thoroughly cooled, then cut into squares. Add millet squares to the bowl with the onion and pickle mixture and mix gently. Serve at room temperature or chilled.

Serves 4.

Millet and Sweet Vegetables

1 cup millet, washed and drained

2½ cups water

Pinch sea salt or 1-inch piece kombu

2 cups diced sweet vegetables (any combination of winter squash, carrots, onions, cabbage, etc.)

Place millet in a large pot with water, salt or kombu, and vegetables. Bring to a boil over high heat, reduce heat to low, cover and cook, uncovered,

35 minutes. Spread cooked millet in a rectangular baking dish and set aside to cool. Cut into squares and serve.

Serves 4–5.

Quinoa and/or Amaranth

Enjoy this as a healthy and tasty breakfast cereal.

2 cups water
1 cup quinoa or amaranth or a combination
¼ cup raisins (optional)
1 pinch salt
1 pinch cinnamon

In a large saucepan, bring water to a boil over high heat. Add quinoa and/or amaranth, raisins (if using), salt, and cinnamon. Return to a boil, cover, and reduce heat to low. Simmer for 20 to 30. Serve hot.

Serves 2–4.

Bulgur

Bulgur is cracked wheat (avoid it if you are sensitive to wheat). It cooks up into a fluffy grain that makes a nice accompaniment for savory meals.

3 cups water
2 cups bulgur
Pinch salt
Thinly sliced scallions or toasted sesame seeds for garnish

In a large saucepan, bring water to a boil over high heat. Add bulgur and salt, cover, and reduce heat to low. Simmer for 20 minutes. Garnish with scallions or sesame seeds and serve hot.

Serves 4–6.

Buckwheat (Kasha)

1 cup white buckwheat groats
2½ cups water

Pinch salt
1 medium onion, diced

Roast buckwheat groats in a skillet over medium heat for 4 to 5 minutes. Place roasted buckwheat in a pot with water, salt, and onions and bring to a boil over high heat. Cover with a tight-fitting lid, reduce heat to medium-low, and simmer for 30 minutes or until all of the water has been absorbed. Stir and serve hot.

Serves 2–4.

Buckwheat and Bows

Cooked buckwheat (see preceding recipe)
1 cup cooked bowtie noodles
Tamari or soy sauce to taste

Combine cooked buckwheat and noodles, add tamari or soy sauce to taste, and serve hot.

Serves 2–4.

Polenta

For dinner, serve polenta garnished with toasted sunflower or sesame seeds. For a sweet hot breakfast, add maple or brown rice syrup.

3 cups water
1 cup cornmeal (may be dry-roasted for a nuttier flavor), mixed with
    one cup water
Pinch salt

Bring water to a boil over high heat. Whisk in the cornmeal-water mixture, add salt and return to a boil, stirring continually to prevent clumping. Lower heat to medium-low and simmer for 30 to 45 minutes, depending on how coarsely ground your cornmeal is.

Serves 4.

Millet and Cauliflower

½ head of cauliflower, cut into small pieces

1 cup millet, washed and drained

4 cups water

2 pinches salt

Chopped fresh parsley, sliced scallions, or roasted seeds for garnish

Place cauliflower in the bottom of a large pot, top with the millet, and gently pour the water into one side of the pot to keep the layering intact. Add salt and cover. Bring to a rapid boil over high heat, reduce heat to medium-low, and simmer for 45 minutes or longer, until grain is tender. Stir from the bottom to the top of the pot. Garnish with chopped parsley, sliced scallions, or roasted seeds.

Serves 4–6.

Sweet Rice Porridge

1 cup sweet brown rice, washed

5 cups water

Pinch sea salt

¼ cup raisins

¼ cup dried peaches, pears or apricots, soaked and diced

¼ cup dried apple, soaked and diced

Place all ingredients in a large pot, cover, and bring to a boil over high heat. Reduce heat to low and cook for 50 minutes or longer, until rice is tender. Remove from heat and allow to cool. Serve warm.

Serves 4.

Udon Noodles in Broth

6 cups water

1 8-ounce package of udon (or brown rice) noodles

1 strip kombu

2 shiitake mushrooms, halved and with stem ends removed

1 tablespoon soy sauce

2–4 tablespoons bonito fish flakes

1 tablespoon grated fresh ginger

3 scallions, thinly sliced

In a large pot, bring the water to a rapid boil. Add noodles, kombu, mushrooms, soy sauce, fish flakes, and grated ginger and cook, uncovered, for 15 to 25 minutes or until noodles are soft. Serve hot, garnished with scallions.
    Serves 4.

Spiral Noodles

3 tablespoons olive oil

1 onion, diced

10 button mushrooms, diced

10 cups spinach, cut small

5 sun-dried tomatoes, soaked for twenty minutes and cut into small pieces

3 cups cooked spiral noodles

Tamari or soy sauce to taste

Handful of pinenuts for garnish

In a large skillet, heat olive oil over medium-high heat. Add onion, mushrooms, spinach, and sun-dried tomatoes and cook, covered, until vegetables are soft. Add water if necessary. When vegetables are soft, add noodles and stir in tamari or soy sauce to taste. Garnish with pinenuts and serve hot.
    Serves 4.

Soba Noodles with Sauce

½ pound soba noodles

¼ cup tamari or soy sauce

2 tablespoons unrefined sesame oil

1 tablespoon toasted sesame oil

1 tablespoon brown rice vinegar

2 teaspoons maple syrup

1 teaspoon finely grated fresh ginger

1 teaspoon chopped garlic

1 cup chopped scallions

1 tablespoon toasted sesame seeds

Cook soba noodles in boiling water until soft. Drain and rinse thoroughly with cold water. In a small bowl, combine tamari or soy sauce, oils, vinegar, maple syrup, ginger, and garlic. Pour mixture over noodles, add scallions and seeds, and toss to mix.

Serves 3.

Noodle Salad

½ pound tofu

1 tablespoon sesame tahini

2 tablespoons light miso (such as Westbrae Organic Mellow White Miso)

1 tablespoon lemon juice

¼ cup water

2 cups cooked noodles

½ cup diced carrots, cooked in boiling water for two minutes and drained

½ cup peas, cooked in boiling water for two minutes and drained

½ cup corn kernels, cooked in boiling water for two minutes and drained

¼ cup sliced scallions

1 tablespoon roasted sesame seeds

In blender or food processor, combine the tofu, tahini, miso, lemon juice, and water and process until smooth.

In a large bowl, combine the cooked noodles and vegetables. Toss with the dressing until well combined. Garnish with scallions and sesame seeds.

Serves 4–6.

Vegetables

Sautéed Leafy Greens

1 bunch leafy greens, cut into ½-inch strips

2–3 tablespoons olive or macadamia nut oil

Tamari or soy sauce to taste

In a large skillet, heat oil over medium-high heat and add greens. Cook, stirring gently, until the greens begin to change color. Cover and simmer for 2 minutes. Add tamari or soy sauce and a little water, if necessary, to complete cooking.

Serves 4.

Steamed Vegetables

1 bunch leafy greens, cut into ½-inch strips
Pinch sea salt
Toasted sesame oil, tamari or soy sauce, and/or umeboshi vinegar to taste

Place greens in a large pot with one inch of water, cover, and bring to a boil. Cook for 2 minutes. Remove greens from water and season with toasted sesame oil, tamari or soy sauce, and/or umeboshi vinegar as desired.

Serves 3–4.

Herbed Parsnips

2 medium parsnips, cut on the diagonal into ½-inch rounds
1 teaspoon walnut, almond, or olive oil
⅓ cup fresh parsley
2 teaspoons minced fresh thyme leaves or ½ teaspoon dried
1½ teaspoons fresh lemon juice
Shoyu soy sauce to taste

In a large pot, steam parsnips over boiling water for 5 to 10 minutes, or until tender. In a medium bowl, combine oil, parsley, thyme, and lemon juice. Add hot parsnips and toss with oil-herb mixture. Season with shoyu soy sauce to taste and serve.

Serves 2–3.

Carrot and Raisin Salad

Carrots, grated
Raisins
Sea salt to taste
Gingered Vinaigrette Dressing (see recipe, pages 241–242), optional

In a large bowl, combine grated carrots, raisins, and salt. Place a plate directly on top of the vegetables and place a heavy weight, such as a jug of water, a brick, or a heavy rock, on top of the plate and press for at least 30 minutes and up to 60 minutes. Rinse well and drain. Serve plain or tossed with the vinaigrette.

Sautéed Vegetables with Sweet and Sour Sauce

4 ounces Chinese cabbage, thinly sliced on the diagonal

4 ounces carrots, cut into thin flowers

4 ounces lotus root, cut into matchstick-sized pieces

4 ounces kale, thinly sliced

4 ounces yellow squash, cut into matchstick-sized pieces

4 ounces mushrooms, thinly sliced

½ cup apple juice

1 tablespoon shoyu soy sauce

2 tablespoons rice vinegar

1–2 tablespoons kuzu mixed with 2 ounces cold water

Sprouts for garnish

In a large skillet, heat a small amount of water over high heat. Add the cabbage, carrots, lotus root, kale, squash, and mushrooms and sauté until the vegetables are tender, yet crisp, and still retain their bright colors.

In a saucepan, combine the apple juice, shoyu soy sauce, rice vinegar, and diluted kuzu and bring to a simmer over medium heat. Cook just until sauce begins to thicken and becomes clear.

Pour hot sauce over sautéed vegetables and mix to coat all vegetables. Garnish with sprouts and serve.

Serves 4.

Tofu, Mushrooms, and Kale

1½ cups almonds

¼ cup plus 2–3 tablespoons shoyu soy sauce

1 cup water

3 cloves garlic

2 pounds tofu, diced

1 quart mushrooms, sliced

2 cups onions, diced

2 tablespoons sesame oil

1 teaspoon sea salt

2 tablespoons chopped fresh thyme

2 tablespoons chopped fresh basil

1 large bunch kale, chopped

Preheat oven to 350° F.

Spread almonds on a baking sheet and bake in preheated oven for approximately 10 minutes until lightly browned. Toss almonds with 2 to 3 tablespoons shoyu soy sauce and set aside to cool. When cool, place in a food processor with water and garlic and puree until smooth.

In a large skillet, heat oil over medium-high heat. Add tofu, mushrooms, and onions and sauté for 5 to 10 minutes. Add the remaining ¼ cup shoyu soy sauce, thyme, basil, and kale. Simmer for another 10 minutes, or until the kale is tender.

Serves 4.

Boiled Vegetable Salad with Pumpkinseed Dressing

Chinese cabbage, sliced in thin diagonals

Kale, thinly sliced

Daikon radish, cut into matchstick-sized pieces

Scallions, cut into 3-inch lengths

Pumpkinseed Dressing (see recipe, page 242)

Bring a large pot with 2 to 3 inches of water in it to a boil. Add Chinese cabbage and cook for 45 seconds. Remove cabbage from pot, and drain. Next add kale, cook for 60 seconds, remove from pot, and drain. Follow with the daikon for 60 seconds, and finally, scallions for 5 seconds. The vegetables should be tender, yet retain their bright colors. Arrange vegetables on a serving platter, drizzle with the Pumpkinseed Dressing, and serve.

Corn Salad with Creamy Tofu-Dill Dressing

2 cups fresh sweet corn kernels
½ cup fresh green beans, cut into 1-inch lengths
¼ cup red onion, diced
¼ cup grated carrot
1 cup shredded lettuce
Creamy Tofu-Dill Dressing (see recipe, page 241)

Place 2 to 3 inches of water in a large pot and bring to a boil over high heat. Blanch the corn for 2 minutes, drain and set aside. Next, blanch the green beans for 2 to 3 minutes, drain and combine with the corn in a large bowl. Add the red onion, carrots, and lettuce and toss to mix. Spoon dressing over each serving of salad just before serving.

Serves 3–4.

Baked Winter Squash

1 large acorn squash (or any winter variety), washed, cut in half, and seeded

Preheat oven 350° to 375°F.

Place the squash halves on a cookie sheet, cut side down. Bake in preheated oven at for about 1 hour, until soft all the way through when a fork is inserted in the center. Serve hot.

Serves 4.

Root Vegetable Stew

2 strips kombu
1 burdock stalk, sliced
1 onion, cut into chunks
2 carrots, cut into chunks
1 winter squash, cut into chunks
¼–½ teaspoon salt

Preheat oven to 350°F.

In a baking dish, layer kombu, burdock, onion, carrots, and squash.

Add ½ inch water and sprinkle with salt. Cover and bake in preheated oven for 1 hour, or until vegetables are soft.

Serves 4.

Cucumber, Wakame, and Watercress Salad

1 tablespoon toasted sesame oil

6 tablespoons brown rice vinegar

3 tablespoons tamari or soy sauce

1½ tablespoons water

1 4-inch piece wakame, simmered in water for 15 minutes, drained, and cut into small pieces

3 cucumbers, julienned

3 bunches watercress, chopped

In a small bowl, combine oil, vinegar, tamari or soy sauce, and water. In a medium bowl combine the wakame, cucumber, and watercress. Add the sauce to the vegetables and toss until well combined.

Serves 3.

Chinese-Style Vegetables

The thinner you cut the vegetables, the quicker they will cook. Feel free to add canned baby corn, water chestnuts, or diced tofu.

3 tablespoons sesame oil

½ cup carrots, cut into matchstick-sized pieces

½ cup thinly sliced celery

½ cup trimmed snow peas

½ cup thinly sliced mushrooms

1 tablespoon soy sauce

1 tablespoon arrowroot flour, dissolved in 1/4 cup water

1 cup bean sprouts

In a large skillet, heat oil over high heat. When oil is hot, add the vegetables one at a time, starting with carrots, then adding the celery, snow peas, and mushrooms. Sauté over high heat, stirring frequently, until vegetables are soft. Add soy sauce and arrowroot mixture. Gently mix in bean sprouts. Serve hot.

Serves 4.

Beans

Vegetable Tofu Cream Cheese

Use this tangy spread as a substitute for cream cheese.

1 pound fresh tofu
2¼ teaspoons umeboshi paste
½ teaspoon tahini
1½ tablespoons chopped scallion
½ stalk celery, minced
¼ teaspoon chopped parsley
½ medium carrot, grated

Steam tofu in two inches of water in a covered pot for 2 minutes. Remove immediately. Crumble tofu into a blender, add umeboshi paste and tahini, and blend, adding only enough water to create a creamy texture.

In medium bowl, combine vegetables. Add the tofu mixture and stir briefly, just to mix.

Serves 4.

Vegetarian Chili

Canned beans may be substituted here. Simply skip the step of cooking the beans with the bay leaf before adding the other ingredients.

1 cup dried kidney beans, soaked 6–8 hours or overnight
1 cup dried pinto beans, soaked 6–8 hours or overnight
2-inch piece kombu
1 bay leaf
1 medium onion, diced
2 cloves garlic, minced
½ teaspoon oregano
¼ teaspoon sea salt

½ teaspoon cayenne pepper or chili powder (optional)
Bulgur wheat (quinoa or amaranth can be substituted)
Minced parsley for garnish

Drain soaked beans and place in a large pot with five to six cups of fresh water. Bring to a boil and cook, uncovered, for 5 minutes. Add kombu and bay leaf, cover, reduce heat to low and cook for 90 minutes or longer, until the beans are tender.

When beans are done, remove bay leaf and add onion, garlic, oregano, salt, cayenne or chili powder (if using), and bulgur. Continue to cook, covered, until onions are soft, about 10 to 15 minutes more. Garnish with parsley.

Serves 4–6.

Tempeh Patties

8 ounces tempeh, cut into 2-inch pieces
2 tablespoons flour
2 tablespoons water
½ teaspoon dried sage
½ teaspoon dried thyme
½ teaspoon dried rosemary
1½ tablespoons shoyu soy sauce
2 cloves garlic, minced
2 teaspoons sesame oil

Steam tempeh over boiling water for 10 minutes. In a bowl, mash tempeh and mix with flour, water, sage, thyme, rosemary, shoyu, and garlic. Form mixture into 4 patties. Heat oil in skillet, add patties, and fry until golden on both sides. Tempeh patties can be served with a grain and vegetables for a delicious dinner or served on sourdough bread with lettuce, onion, and mustard for a satisfying lunch.

Serves 3–4.

Marinated Chickpea Salad

¼ cup organic sesame or extra virgin olive oil
2–3 tablespoons umeboshi vinegar

2 cups cooked chickpeas
1 small cucumber, quartered and sliced
4 red radishes, sliced in half moons
2 stalks celery, diced
¼ cup minced parsley
Sprouts or lettuce for garnish

In a medium bowl, combine the oil and vinegar. Add the chickpeas and stir to coat. Refrigerate, covered, for at least 1 to 2 hours and as long as a full day.

An hour before serving, add cucumber, radishes, and celery to the chickpeas. Just before serving, stir in parsley. On a serving platter, place a layer of lettuce leaves or sprouts and place the chickpea salad on top. Serve with pita bread.

Serves 4.

Black Beans with Onions, Carrots, and Peppers

Canned beans may be substituted. Simply omit the first step of cooking the beans.

2 cups dried black beans, rinsed, drained, and soaked overnight
1 strip kombu
1 large onion, diced
1 large carrot, diced
1 green bell pepper, diced
Miso to taste

Place beans in a large pot covered with fresh water. Add kombu and bring to a boil over high heat. Reduce heat to medium-low and simmer, covered, for about 2 hours, or until beans are tender. Add the onion, carrot, and bell pepper and simmer another 20 minutes. Add miso during last few minutes of cooking.

Serves 4.

Lentils with Onion, Winter Squash, and Kombu

French lentils are the smallest and therefore, the quickest to cook.

1 cup lentils, rinsed and drained
8 cups water
1 strip kombu
1 onion, diced
1 cup diced winter squash
Tamari or soy sauce to taste

Place the lentils in a large pot with the water and kombu and bring to a boil over high heat. Reduce heat to medium and cook for 1 hour. Add onion, squash, and tamari or soy sauce and cook about 30 minutes more, until vegetables are soft.

Serves 3.

Sweet Pinto Beans

2 cups dried pinto beans, soaked overnight
1 strip kombu
4 cups water
2–4 ounces miso
4 ounces apple butter

Place beans and kombu in a large pot with the water and bring to a boil over high heat. Reduce heat to medium and cook for 2 hours.

Preheat oven to 350ºF.

In a small bowl, combine miso and apple butter and stir into beans. Place bean mixture into a baking dish and bake in preheated oven for 30 minutes.

Serves 4.

Scrambled Tofu

1 tablespoon olive oil
3 scallions, thinly sliced
1 pound tofu, mashed

⅛ teaspoon turmeric

1 tablespoon soy sauce

Heat oil in a frying pan over high heat, add scallions, and sauté for 1 minute. Add tofu and turmeric and continue to cook, stirring frequently, for 5 minutes. Add soy sauce and cook until the liquid has evaporated.

Serves 2–3.

Tofu with Tamari and Ginger

1 pound organic tofu, cut into large chunks (or the same quantity of cooked beans)

A few drops of tamari

One teaspoon grated ginger

Sliced scallions for garnish

Place tofu in a large pot and add water to cover. Bring to boil over high heat, add tamari and grated ginger, and reduce heat to medium. Cook until the water is almost gone. Garnish with sliced scallions. Serves 4.

Tempeh with Sauerkraut

1 tablespoon olive oil

1 pound of tempeh, diced

½ medium cabbage, thinly sliced

½ cup sauerkraut (natural, organic, "live")

1 cup water

½ teaspoon light miso dissolved in 1 tablespoon water

¼ cup thinly sliced scallions

Heat oil in frying pan and brown the tempeh evenly on both sides. Add cabbage and sauté with tempeh for 5 minutes. Place the sauerkraut on top, add the water, cover, and steam for 20 minutes. Stir in the miso mixture and simmer for 5 minutes. Mix in the scallions.

Serves 4.

Sea Vegetables

Arame with Lemon and Sesame Seeds

1 package arame seaweed

1 tablespoon soy sauce

1 teaspoon grated lemon zest

½ cup ground roasted sesame seeds

Lemon wedges and scallions for garnish

Rinse arame in a strainer under running water. Place arame in a pot with enough water to cover and let sit for 3 to 5 minutes. Bring to a boil over high heat, cover, reduce the heat to medium-low, and simmer for 10 minutes. Remove the lid, add the soy sauce, and boil until all the liquid has evaporated. Add the lemon zest and sesame seeds and mix well. Serve with lemon wedges and garnish with fresh sliced scallions.

Serves 4.

Fish

Broiled Fish

1 pound firm-fleshed white fish

½ cup water

¼ teaspoon soy sauce

½ teaspoon ginger juice

Wash fish under cold water. In a medium bowl, combine water, soy sauce, and ginger juice. Add the fish, turning to coat, and marinate in the refrigerator for 1 hour.

Place fish on an oiled baking sheet under the broiler, and broil for about 5 to 8 minutes, depending on the size and thickness of the fish, on each side until cooked through.

Serves 4.

Whitefish Salad

1 pound firm-fleshed white fish

1 cup diced celery

1 cup sliced scallions

1 tablespoon Nayonnaise*

3 whole-grain rolls, sliced tomatoes, and lettuce for serving

Steam fish, covered, in small amount of water until tender. Remove from heat and drain. In a medium bowl, flake fish with a fork and combine with celery, scallions, and Nayonnaise. Serve on rolls with sandwich fixings. *Tofu mayonnaise available at most natural foods stores.

Serves 3.

Fish Soup

½- to ¾-pound firm-fleshed white fish fillet

6–8 cups water

1 strip kombu, soaked and cut into thin strips

1 teaspoon salt

2 cups thinly sliced leeks

1 cup bite-sized pieces Chinese cabbage

1 cup diced carrot

1 tablespoon soy sauce

¼ teaspoon freshly grated ginger

Chopped parsley for garnish

Rinse fish quickly under cold running water and cut into small pieces. Bring the water and kombu to a boil in a saucepan set over high heat, add the fish and salt, cover, reduce heat to low, and simmer for 25 minutes. Add leeks, cabbage, and carrot and return to a boil over high heat. Reduce heat to low and simmer for 5 minutes. Add soy sauce and grated ginger and simmer for 2 minutes more. Stir with a wooden spoon to mix the vegetables and fish evenly. Garnish with chopped parsley.

Serves 6.

Sauces and Dressings

Sesame Seed and Scallion Condiment

1 cup diced onion

1 cup diced red pepper

1 cup sliced scallions

1 tablespoon miso

1 cup sesame seeds

Sauté onion, red pepper, and scallions in olive oil over medium-high heat until tender. Add miso and cook a few minutes longer. Toss with sesame seeds and use as a condiment on grains.

Creamy Tofu-Dill Dressing

½ pound firm tofu (or substitute ½ pound of beans)

¼ cup water

2 tablespoons umeboshi vinegar

½ teaspoon shoyu soy sauce

¼ cup chopped fresh dill

Place tofu, water, umeboshi vinegar, rice vinegar, shoyu, and dill in a blender and puree until smooth and creamy.

Vinaigrette Dressing

4 tablespoons toasted sesame oil

4 tablespoons tamari or soy sauce

Juice of ½ lemon

Combine sesame oil, tamari or soy sauce, and lemon juice in a covered jar and shake. Toss with salads or greens.

Gingered Vinaigrette Dressing

1 tablespoon brown rice vinegar

½ teaspoon fresh ginger juice

½ teaspoon sea salt

In a small saucepan, combine the vinegar, ginger juice, and salt. Bring to a simmer over medium heat and cook for 1 to 2 minutes. Let cool and toss with salads or leafy greens.

Orange-Miso Dressing

¼ cup freshly squeezed orange juice

1–1½ teaspoons white miso

1 tablespoon ground roasted sesame seeds (optional)

In a small bowl, cream miso with orange juice until smooth. Mix in sesame seeds (if using). Toss with salads or leafy greens.

Pumpkinseed Dressing

1 cup pumpkinseeds

1 teaspoon umeboshi paste

2-3 teaspoons brown rice syrup

1 teaspoon lemon juice (optional)

1½–1 cup water

Roast the pumpkinseeds in a skillet over high heat, then grind in a suribachi (a Japanese-style pestle that uses a mortar called a surikoji). In a small bowl, combine ground seeds with umeboshi paste, brown rice syrup, lemon juice (if using), and half of the water. Mix well, taste, and add the rest of the water if a thinner consistency is desired.

Serves 4.

Desserts

Kanten

1 quart apple or other unsweetened fruit juice

Pinch salt

½ teaspoon vanilla extract (optional)

⅓ cup agar flakes

1 tablespoon arrowroot or kuzu dissolved in ¼ cup apple juice

1 pint strawberries, quartered

Combine apple juice, salt, vanilla extract (if using), and agar flakes in a saucepan and bring to a boil, stirring constantly. Whisk in the arrowroot or kuzu mixture and continue stirring until the mixture returns to a boil. Reduce the heat to medium-low and simmer for 5 minutes. Rinse a square glass pan or bowl with cold water, place the strawberries in the pan, and pour the hot apple juice mixture over the fruit. Chill in the refrigerator until set, approximately 1 hour.

Serves 5–6.

Strawberry Mousse

5 cups apple juice
Pinch sea salt
4 tablespoons agar flakes
2 cups sliced strawberries
2 peaches (or pears or apples), thinly sliced
4 tablespoons kuzu powder
2 teaspoons lime juice (optional)

In a large pot, combine the apple juice, sea salt, and agar flakes and bring to a boil over high heat. Reduce heat to medium-low and simmer for 5 to 10 minutes, until the agar flakes are dissolved. Add the strawberries and peaches or other fruit. Dissolve kuzu in four tablespoons of the hot juice and add to the pot. Cook, stirring constantly, for 1 to 2 minutes. Stir in lime juice (if using). Cool to room temperature or refrigerate until set. Serve as is or put in the blender for lighter dessert.
Serves 4.

Amasake Fruit Smoothies

1 quart amasake
1 quart strawberries, blueberries, or other fresh fruit of your choice
Rice syrup (optional)
Fresh mint for garnish

Place amasake and fruit into a blender and puree as is or, if desired, add a few ice cubes. Add rice syrup (if using) to taste. Garnish with a mint sprig and serve cold with a straw.

Rice Pudding

Leftover white basmati rice, sushi rice, or brown rice

Amasake, enough to make the rice creamy

Brown rice syrup (to taste)

Vanilla extract (to taste)

Raisins (optional)

Grated lemon or orange rind (to taste)

Combine all ingredients in a pot and simmer until soft and creamy. Spoon into individual serving bowls and garnish with fresh fruit or toasted nuts, if desired.

Serves 4.

Coffee Gelatin

4 cups apple juice

2½ tablespoons grain coffee

⅓ cup agar flakes

2 tablespoons tahini

¼ teaspoon cinnamon

⅛ teaspoon salt

Whip all ingredients together in a blender, pour into a saucepan set over high heat, and bring to a boil. Reduce heat to medium-low and simmer for 5 minutes. Rinse a bowl with cold water, add the hot apple juice mixture, and chill in the refrigerator until set, approximately 1 hour.

Serves 6.

For more excellent cooking guidance, I recommend *The Self Healing Cookbook,* by Kristina Turner, and *Macrobiotic Cooking for Everyone,* by Aveline Kushi and Wendy Esko. You'll also find more recipes on our website at www.thepmc.org.

Appendix

The following documents will prove valuable in your journey to improved health. I have included a list of Wellness Protection and Disease Prevention Goals that you can use as a handy guide and general standard to follow in meeting your health objectives. The Food Mantra table contains whole and unprocessed food suggestions that are correct for our human biology. These include grains, vegetables, and beans (GVB); and fruit, nuts, seeds, and wild game (if desired). I also recommend filling out the 7-Day Diet Record to bring to light your true eating habits. It will be helpful to then compare your recorded food choices to the recommendations laid out in the Food Mantra table. If you record everything that you eat and drink for seven days you will see clearly what you need to change in your diet. Perhaps you struggle with impulsive eating. The article "Overcoming Impulsivity" addresses this issue and offers some ideas for conquering this problem. My letter regarding healthy cholesterol levels that was published in the *American Journal of Cardiology* may also be of interest to you.

These documents have been selected from several that are given to every new patient who comes to my practice with the purpose of helping to prevent "virtually all diseases simultaneously." I hope these will be a genuine help to you.

Wellness Protection and Disease Prevention Goals ("Numbers" and Insights)

(For the generally well and modified appropriately for those with health issues)

The following results are ideal numbers and indicators of good health. These can be performed at most medical laboratories. The diet and lifestyle goals are tips for improving your health.

Laboratory Test Results

1. **Non-HDL cholesterol** (is ALL of the "bad cholesterol." To find this number, subtract the "good" HDL cholesterol from the total cholesterol): goal lower than 90.
2. **Triglycerides** (similar in effect to cholesterol): goal lower than 100.
3. **Lp (a)** (similar in effect to cholesterol): goal 15 or lower.
4. **Homocysteine** (similar in effect to cholesterol): goal 7 or lower.
5. **A1C diabetes test:** 5.5 or lower at age 55.
6. **Blood sugar:** 90 at 90 minutes after a meal.
7. **Cardiac HS CRP** (body inflammation test, similar in effect to high cholesterol): 1.0 or lower.
8. **Blood Pressure:** 110/60 or so.
9. **Body Fat Percent** (manifested as "clear lines of definition/demarcation on the abdomen" (CLOD/D), meaning that you can see where the muscles meet the muscles): 11–22 percent for men, 15–27 percent for women.
10. **Uric Acid** (associated with high blood pressure, kidney stones): goal 5.5 or lower.
11. **BUN** (kidney test): 12 or less.
12. **Magnesium** (relates to diet and diabetes prevention): 2.1 or higher.
13. **Potassium** (relates to diabetes prevention, high blood pressure, kidneys): 4.1–4.5.
14. **25 hydroxy (OH) vitamin D3** (measure of vitamin D level): 50 +

15. **PSA** (prostate test): 1.0 or lower.
16. **TSH** (thyroid test): 0.35–3.50.
17. **Hemoglobin** (measure of blood thickness): 14 or so.

Diet and Lifestyle Goals

1. If you need to lose weight, avoid eating chicken, turkey, rice, sandwiches, cereal, and much fruit.
2. If you are overweight, keep a diet diary of everything you eat or drink except for tea, cooked vegetables, vegetable soups, and up to eight ounces of beans per day. You'll lose weight if your diary is empty.
3. My healthiest patients are vegan (no eggs, fish, fowl, dairy, or meat)
3. Eat foods (exactly) as they grow in the field: grains, vegetables, beans (GVB), fruit, nuts, and seeds.
4. Live by the Food Mantra: Fresh (fruits and vegetables), Whole and Unprocessed (grains and beans), Organic (all), and Fiber (all) at the 90+ percent level is the goal.
5. **Less than 12 percent sodium** in any one serving that you eat.
6. If you are overweight, start every meal, including breakfast, with cooked vegetables and/or vegetable soups (but omit potatoes, sweet potatoes, yams, plantain, yucca, jicama, and calabaza).
7. In general, eat only out of a bowl; "wrong" foods tend to be served on plates.
8. Learn about and participate in fitness programs that include Aerobic Interval Training, the PACE program, and BLITZing.
9. Smoking is best dealt with by a combination of support and medication including Chantix, Wellbutrin (bupropion), and the nicotine patch/inhaler/gum.
10. Limit alcohol to four six-ounce glasses of wine (or bottles of beer or shots of hard liquor) or less per week.
11. Accept and deal with reality: wishing, wanting, and hoping are like alcohol; only safe in small doses.

12. If you have high blood pressure, purchase an Omron wrist blood pressure cuff; have it validated at your doctor's office; check your blood pressure before, after, and in between meals.
13. Many conditions are vastly improved with 100 percent avoidance of ALL wheat (including rye), dairy, and soy.

The Food Mantra: Fresh (Fruits and Vegetables), Whole and Unprocessed (Grains and Beans), Organic Preferred

Grains	Vegetables	Beans	Fruits, Nuts, and Seeds	Fish
The fewer processed grains, the better. Choose whole grains over grain flours whenever possible.	Fresh vegetables are best, but frozen are acceptable.	Dried, canned, organic, low-sodium, or frozen are preferred.	Fresh fruits are best, but frozen are acceptable.	Choose wild, not farm-raised fish (be sure to ask your fish monger).
Gluten-free grains: millet (low-fat), quinoa (low-fat, quick-cooking, good for the heart), amaranth (quick-cooking, high protein), teff (quick cooking), and brown rice (promotes weight stability).	Collard greens Broccoli Cauliflower Carrots Winter squash Onions Mushrooms Cabbage	Lentils, mung, aduki, split peas, and black-eyed peas (these are less likely to cause gas than other beans). Gas is reduced by soaking beans with the probiotic L. casei.	Berries or plums (try them cooked in 1 inch of apple, peach, or pear juice, or Rice Dream Vanilla Enriched drink and serve warm).	**Serving sizes:** If you are trim and athletic you may have a palm-sized serving 2 or 3 times per week (you may substitute bison, free-range chicken, or cage-free eggs for fish). If overweight, limit fish to one serving every 14 days.
Grains cause weight gain/inhibit weight loss as do breads, cereals, pasta, potatoes, and oat groats (whole oats).	Celery Bok choy Daikon Kale Leeks	Lima, navy, great northern beans, and chickpeas (these are healthy choices, but more likely to cause gas than the beans listed above). See above regarding soaking.	Cantaloupe, honeydew, and watermelon. Nuts, seeds, sea vegetables, miso, and tamari.	**Choose low-mercury fish:** white fish, freshwater trout, sardines, wild Alaskan salmon, pacific oysters, orange roughy, shrimp, and scallops.
Grains containing gluten: barley (great for muscle development). Wheat and rye berries are highly allergenic.	Scallions Cucumbers Green beans Mustard greens Burdock	Tempeh: Some ingredients to add flavor include balsamic vinegar (Fini Brand), mirin sweet rice cooking wine, oregano, garlic, cilantro, Mrs. Dash, or Spike.	**These fruits inhibit weight loss/cause weight gain (but are okay for those at their proper weight):** apples, pears, peaches, cherries, and grapes.	**Medium-mercury should be eaten only once in a while:** saltwater trout, flounder, lobster, halibut, snapper, cod, haddock, ocean and freshwater perch, sole, and bluefish
Buckwheat (kasha) is high in calcium.	**These are reputed to cause arthritis:** potatoes, sweet potatoes, yams, plantains, eggplant, zucchini, tomatoes, peppers, and spinach.	Beans are perfect proteins: start adapting to them by having just 1 teaspoon a day.	**In general, avoid:** tropical fruits such as bananas, oranges, and pineapples unless you live in the tropics. Eating local produce is believed to be best.	**Avoid high-mercury fish:** Chilean sea bass, grouper, halibut, swordfish, tuna, and amberjack

All grains cook alike: All grains are cooked in boiling water at a ratio of 2:1 (two cups of water to one cup of grain). Cooking times vary by grain, but for all of them, soaking overnight will reduce their cooking time by half. For instance, unsoaked brown rice takes an hour to cook, while brown rice that has been soaked overnight takes only thirty minutes. To cook grains, bring the water to a boil, add the grain, reduce heat to a simmer, cover, and cook for the appropriate length of time. Cook unsoaked brown rice, oat groats, and barley for sixty minutes; soaked for thirty. Unsoaked millet cooks for forty-five minutes; soaked for twenty-two. Quinoa, amaranth, and teff cook in fourteen minutes, or seven minutes when soaked.

Why unprocessed grains? Unprocessed (whole) grains are nutritionally complete, meaning that they retain all of their natural fiber, vitamins, and antioxidants. When grains are made into flour and put into boxes or packages as commercial cereals and breads, the antioxidants such as vitamins C, E, and beta carotene become oxidized and are lost, as is some of the fiber.

DATE: ___ / ___ / ___   NAME: _____

7-Day Diet Record

Day 1	Day 2	Day 3	Day 4	Day 5	Day 6	Day 7

Please list all that you eat or drink except cooked vegetables, vegetable soups, beans, tea, or water. Try not to snack or eat after dinner but tell the truth. Also write in your daily exercise. It would be helpful to review the recommendations included in the Food Mantra table as you work on this. You may photocopy this chart, if that makes it easier to use.

Overcoming Impulsivity

Why do so many of us fail to eat the way we know we should? We know that a diet of cooked vegetables, vegetable soups, and beans is the healthiest way to lose weight and keep it off, yet we continue to give in to our impulses to eat foods we know we shouldn't. Why are we so short-sighted and unmotivated when it comes to planning our meals, and so willing to accept the disease and disability that result from not eating or weighing what we should?

Over-indulging in high-calorie and high-fat foods leads to myriad negative outcomes—high blood pressure, high cholesterol, diabetes, dialysis, stroke, heart attack, dependence on prescription medications, blindness, arthritis, cancer, open-heart surgery, high health care costs, depression, poor self-image, and more—but still we eat poorly and let ourselves remain overweight.

Like it or not, overeating is the main factor causing one to be over-weight (exercise is important, but the real problem is over-indulgence in high-calorie foods like meat, cheese, eggs, butter, cream, oils, rice, bread, waffles, pancakes, cereal, pasta, sweets, soda, fruit, and carbohydrates in general). The way we eat has proven and extreme negative consequences, and yet we regularly disregard this information, succumbing instead to our desire for instant gratification and immediate rewards. Overcoming this "dis-inhibition" and commiting to eating right could save us from dependence on prescription drugs, hospitalizations, surgery, and disease, yet too many of us allow ourselves to be slaves to our impulsive urges.

Impulsivity, or lack of impulse control, is a difficulty in postponing gratification. Often our impulses to eat are caused simply by the desire to overcome boredom. Eating is just something to do, a way to break up the time or provide a diversion from mundane activities or tasks. These are all wrong and counterproductive reasons that result in gaining weight or maintaining a body that is overweight.

Impulsive people tend to have a decreased sensitivity to negative consequences when acting or processing information. In other words, impulsive eating is caused by a lack of behavioral inhibition and a disregard of long-term consequences. Cognitive behavior therapy (CBT) and/or medication can be helpful treatments.

The first step in treatment is learning to become more aware of your own habits and using problem-solving skills—preplanning, hesitating, counting before you eat, keeping a diet journal, thinking the situation through, or talking to a counselor (and yourself)—to clarify and commit to long-term goals. By developing the skills to manage contingencies and deal with the unexpected, you can teach yourself to become less impulsive. With a bit of knowledge about eating right and a commitment to your long-term goals, you can make positive changes and maintain them for the rest of your life.

Moeller, F.G., et al. 2001. Impulsivity in psychiatry. *American Journal of Psychiatry.* 58:1783–1793.

Reader's Comment

National Cholesterol Education Program Adult Treatment Panel-III Guidelines and the Abolition of Symptomatic Coronary Artery Disease

The American Journal of Cardiology, Vol. 91. March 1, 2003

The document below that I wrote is a letter to the editor that was selected to be published in 2003 in the *American Journal of Cardiology,* one of the top cardiology journals in the world. It was chosen because the editor of this journal felt that the points I raised were correct and insightful, and it is still fully relevant. My article was in response to the very confusing and too elevated cholesterol levels recommended by the American College of Cardiology and the American Heart Association in their NCEP ATP Guidelines. The terms "myocardial infarction" and "coronary event" mentioned in the letter mean "heart attack." The sentence that includes "high density lipoprotein ... cytokines" addresses body chemicals that, like elevated cholesterol, contribute to the future development of a heart attack or stroke. "Statins ... fibrates" are medications that reduce cholesterol and/or improve triglycerides.

Regarding the reassessment of the National Cholesterol Education Program Adult Treatment Program-III (NCEP ATP-III) cholesterol guidelines referred to in the article by Ansell and Waters[1] concerning "optimal" low-density lipoprotein (LDL) cholesterol levels, the trend continues toward a more coronary artery disease-free recommendation. To me, the current NCEP ATP-III guidelines are so confusing that, even as a board certified cardiologist, I cannot manage them. In addition, these criteria missed 75 percent of myocardial infarctions occurring before the age of fifty-five years, as reported by Kwame Osei Akosah, MD, at the 2002 Eighth World Congress on Heart Failure. At some levels of blood cholesterol coronary artery disease does not occur. Virtually all pre-technologic societies have a total cholesterol of 90 to 130 mg/dl, with the associated benefit of no known coronary disease (and a vastly decreased incidence of diverticulitis; arthritis; cancer of the colon, prostate, uterus, breast, and so on). Thirty-five percent of coronary events occur with a total cholesterol between 150 to 200 mg/dl.[2] In the Framingham study, Castelli[3] has found that coronary artery disease essentially ceases to exist with a serum total cholesterol less than 150 mg/dl.

It has become increasingly clear that for those with documented atherosclerotic vascular disease (post- myocardial infarction and/or coronary artery disease documented by angiography or coronary ultrasound) or diabetes mellitus, the ideal goal would be total cholesterol of 130 mg/dl. The roles of other risk factors and/or risk predictors, such as high density lipoprotein, interleukin-6, cardiac highly specific C reactive protein, lipoprotein(a), LDL sub-fractions for pattern A or B, oxidized LDL and its antibody, homocysteine, matrix metaloproteinases, adhesion molecules, and other cytokines, are also being elucidated. My own inner-city practice experience, which began thirty years ago, is identical to that of Ornish[4] and Esselstyn.[5] Virtually none of my patients have developed any cardiac ischemic event if their total cholesterol is kept less than 150 mg/dl. If patients do have coronary disease, none have had a repeat cardiac ischemic event of any variety in my series of twenty consecutive and unselected patients. These patients are now twenty plus years after their cardiac procedure, and their total cholesterol is kept under 130 mg/dl (usually with an LDL of equal to or less than 75 mg/dl).

This absence of symptomatic coronary artery disease is accomplished using a very high fiber diet (75 to 100 grams/day of whole, unprocessed, and ideally organic food—much, much higher than is currently recommended) with fish twice a week and anything once in a while, along with statins and/or niacin and/or fibrates and/or thiazolidinediones and/or biguanides when necessary (commonly). Such an approach can (and does in my, Ornish's, and Esselstyn's cases) achieve the abolition of symptomatic myocardial ischemia when a cholesterol level less than 150 mg/dl is achieved for healthy patients and less than 130 mg/dl for those who have documented coronary disease and/or diabetes mellitus.

We should not treat for a decrease in cholesterol-induced atherosclerotic disease, we should be about its absolute prevention, and such is within our grips. It is with these facts and opinions[6,7] that I make the following recommendation. I propose that the NCEP ATP-III guidelines be scrapped because of their complexity, unlearnability, and ineffectiveness because the total prevention of symptomatic coronary artery disease and real preventive cardiology are physical realities as outlined previously when utilizing much simpler markers (serum total cholesterol either less than 150 mg/dl for healthy patients or less than 130 mg/dl for those with myocardial ischemia and/or diabetes).

H. ROBERT SILVERSTEIN, MD
Hartford, Connecticut
October 14, 2002

1. Ansell BJ, Waters DD. Reassessment of national cholesterol education program adult treatment panel-III guidelines: one year later. *Am J Cardiol* 2002; 90:524–525.

2. Castelli WP. The new pathophysiology of coronary artery disease. *Am J Cardiol* 1998; 82:60T–65T.

3. Roberts W. Getting more people on statins. *Am J Cardiol* 2002; 90:683–685.

4. Ornish D, Scherwitz LW, Billings JH, Gould KL, Merritt TA, Sparler S, Armstrong WT, Ports TA, Kirkeeido RL, Hogeboom C, Brand RJ. Intensive lifestyle changes for reversal of coronary heart disease. *JAMA* 1998; 280:2001–2007.

5. Esselstyn CB. Updating a 12-year experience with arrest and reversal therapy for coronary heart disease (an overdue requiem for palliative cardiology). *Am J Cardiol* 1999; 84:339–341.

6. Silverstein HR. Preventing heart disease. *Lancet* 1990; 335:227.

7. Silverstein HR. Coronary artery disease virtually preventable. *Med World News* 1994; 34:17.

Index

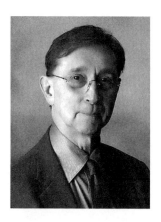

About the Author

Medical director of the Preventive Medicine Center in Hartford, Connecticut, H. Robert Silverstein, MD, FACC, is a board certified cardiologist and internist, and a Fellow of the American Colleges of Preventive Medicine and Cardiology. He is a staff member at Saint Francis and Hartford Hospitals in Connecticut and is a clinical assistant professor of medicine at the University of Connecticut School of Medicine. Due to his interest in alternative medicine, he served on the board of directors for the Connecticut Holistic Health Association (CHHA) and was director of the Hartford chapter for one year. He was voted their outstanding practitioner. He also received an honor for excellence in care of the minority community from the International Society of Hypertension in Blacks (ISHIB). Dr. Silverstein has two cable access television shows, one in West Hartford and the other in Hartford. More information about the author and video links can be found on his website: www.thepmc.org.